Second Edition

HEALTH COMMUNICATION
THEORY & PRACTICE

Gary L. Kreps
Hofstra University

Barbara C. Thornton
University of Nevada, Reno

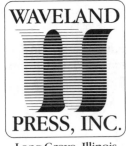

WAVELAND
PRESS, INC.
Long Grove, Illinois

D1167014

Consulting Editor

Robert E. Denton, Jr.

For information about this book, contact:
Waveland Press, Inc.
4180 IL Route 83, Suite 101
Long Grove, IL 60047-9580
(847) 634-0081
info@waveland.com
www.waveland.com

10-digit ISBN 0-88133-643-2
13-digit ISBN 978-0-88133-643-6

Printed in the United States of America

19   18   17

Contents

iii

Chapter

4 Group Communication in Health Care   65

Chapter

5 Organizational Communication in Health Care   91

Preface

This book is about the role of communication in health and health care. We believe that human communication performs an important role in the delivery of health care and the promotion of health. Health care providers depend on their abilities to communicate effectively with their clients and co-workers to accomplish their jobs. Health care consumers depend on their abilities to communicate effectively with health care providers and representatives of the health care system to acquire the best possible health care. Health care system administrators also depend on their abilities to communicate effectively with both health care employees and consumers to coordinate the provision of health care services. In fact, we contend that all people depend on their abilities to communicate to maintain their health and to help others maintain health.

Yet, human communication, for all of its obvious importance, is often ignored and taken for granted within the health care system. Most people assume that since they communicate all the time, communicating is simple. While it is true that we do communicate all the time, it is also true that we often communicate ineffectively. We don't always understand others as well as we could; they probably don't understand us very well either. A great deal of relevant information that might be of use to us is never received or utilized because of deficiencies in human communication. Our purpose in writing this book is to help you recognize the importance of communication in health care, to understand the many ways effective communication can be used to promote health, and to enhance your abilities to communicate effectively within the health care system.

The first edition of *Health Communication* was written almost a decade ago. A great deal of new information about the role of communication in health care is now available. While many of the concepts that were important in the first edition (developing effective provider/consumer relationships, health care teams, and health care interviews) are still important and are presented here, we have included many new concepts in the second edition. We take much stronger positions on the use of communication to promote health, the important role of information in health care, the development of health communication campaigns, the promotion of ethical health communication, and the use of new health communication technologies than we took in the first edition. We provide more balanced coverage about communication issues of concern to both health care providers and consumers. We also provide greater depth of information throughout this edition of the book, reflecting the growth and maturation of health communication research and theory over the past decade.

We take a pragmatic perspective on communication in health care, relating communication research and theory to realistic health care situations. A broad spectrum of research on health and communication is integrated and applied to the many issues facing modern health care providers and consumers in the delivery of health care. Although the book avoids simplistic "cookie cutter" solutions to complex human problems, it does offer insights and strategies which providers and consumers can use to analyze and cope with difficult health communication situations. Human communication is complex and multi-faceted, and certainly there is never one "right" way to communicate in any health care situation. However, this book should help you to develop an appreciation for the many factors influencing human behavior and interaction.

It is our strong contention that in order to solve health communication problems, the study of communication should ideally be interdisciplinary. That is, health care consumers and different members of the health care professions should study communication together to increase interprofessional sensitivity and cooperation. Since it is not always possible to study together, we have designed this book to fill many interdisciplinary needs and to be a bridge between consumers and the many different health care providers. The case histories that are integrated into each chapter describe a wide range of health care situations.

The book is divided into nine major chapters. The first chapter explicates the boundaries of health communication. Current issues in health communication delivery are discussed in light of the impact of human communication on their causes and potential solutions. Chapter 2 examines several important theoretical bases and concepts of human communication relevant to the delivery of health care, providing the reader with a strong theoretical base for the study of health communication. Chapter 3 identifies and explores the interpersonal contexts in which health communication occurs, examining topics such as developing and maintaining effective health care relationships, health care interviewing, and therapeutic communication. Chapter 4 examines the group communication context of health care, focusing on health care teams, ethics committees, self-help groups, conflict maintenance, decision making, and problem solving. Chapter 5 deals with the organizational context of health communication and reviews information on health care delivery systems, as well as problems in coping with modern health care bureaucracies. Chapter 6 explores the development of effective health communication messages in health education and the use of communication media in the modern health care system. Chapter 7 describes the influences of culture on health care and the sensitive use of communication to promote intercultural understanding and cooperation in health care. Chapter 8 examines many complex ethical issues in modern health care and describes the role of human communication in promoting ethical decision making and behavior. The final chapter reviews the role of communication in health promotion and describes strategies for using communication to promote public health.

In writing this book we have paid special attention to using language clearly and sensitively. We have attempted to demystify complex jargon by providing explanations and examples to flesh out and illustrate new and often complex concepts. We have chosen to include both the male and female pronoun when describing health care providers and clients to avoid sexist language usage and sexist stereotypes. On the advice of some of our students, we have decided to limit our use of the connotatively passive term "patients" to describe people who seek health care, opting for the more assertive terms "consumers" and "clients." Throughout the book we attempt to encourage consumer participation in the health care process; using the term client rather than patient can help empower health care consumers.

Writing this book was a collaborative effort and the order of authorship is alphabetical. Barbara Thornton took primary responsibility for writing chapters 1, 3, 4, 7, and 8, and Gary Kreps took primary responsibility for writing chapters 2, 5, 6, and 9, although both authors' ideas and revisions appear throughout the book.

A separate collection of readings is also available to be used in conjunction with this textbook. The readings represent different health care consumer and provider perspectives. The readings are excellent discussion starters for classes and training groups, allowing both students and professionals to integrate and expand upon health communication concepts.

We commissioned several esteemed colleagues, Deborah Ballard Reisch, Lee Ann Glass, Greg Hayes, Trudy Larson, Edward Maibach, Rosalie

Marinelli, and Dorothy Rasinski, to work with us in preparing specific readings that provide coverage of important health communication issues. We also selected several new readings from the best published work available to complement each chapter.

Several people have been of great service to us in writing this book. We are especially indebted to Neil and Carol Rowe of Waveland Press for their eagerness to publish a second edition of this book, as well as for their patience and cooperation. Colleagues and students who used the first edition of the book provided us with insightful feedback and suggestions for revision. Laurie Albright read the entire book and provided excellent suggestions for editing. Our families were patient and understanding with us when we neglected them to complete this book. Tren Anderson, former Executive Editor of College Publishing at Longman Inc., had the foresight to publish the first edition of the book, as well as the wisdom to encourage Neil and Carol to publish the second edition. We miss you Tren and are richer for the time we spent with you. Barbara dedicates this book to her mother, Margery Cavanaugh, and Gary dedicates this book to his mother, Rhoda Cohen Kreps. Thank you all. Gesundheit!

Communication in Health Care

The young woman needed four wisdom teeth extracted. The procedure was a routine one that could be performed in the dentist's office. Nitrous oxide was administered as an anesthetic. The woman's mother accompanied her but was directed to sit in the waiting room, with the promise that she would be called if needed. During the course of the treatment, the woman had a drug reaction. She began to experience terror and wanted her mother. The client tried to ask for her mother, only to find that she was unable to talk. Feeling helpless only increased her terror.

At no time during the one-hour dental procedure did the dentist or the dental assistant inquire into the client's comfort. After the procedure, the client had several psychological reactions, including nightmares which persisted for several months. Today, almost six years later, she continues to feel aversion toward dentists. The dentist and his assistant, questioned by the parent as to why they had not inquired

*into the client's comfort, explained that they typically become so
involved in the procedure that they often do not inquire; also, they
felt at a loss as to how they should approach the client during a
procedure.*

Many similar stories can be told about inadequate communication with
clients who are experiencing pain or fright. However, health professionals
(with rare exceptions) perceive themselves to be helpful and altruistically
motivated persons. How does the communication disparity between "intent"
and "execution" occur? (Thornton, Page & Dangott, 1982).

The Communicative Demands of Health Care Practice

Health communication is an area of study concerned with human interaction in the health care process. It is the way we seek, process and share
health information. Human communication is the singularly most important
tool health professionals have to provide health care to their clients. Not
only do health care providers offer their services to consumers through
communication contact, but they also gather pertinent information from
their clients, explain procedures and regimens to clients, and elicit cooperation among members of their health care team through their ability to
communicate. The processes and theories which explain this communication
are discussed in chapter 2.

Health care professionals depend on their abilities to communicate
effectively with their colleagues, clients, and often the families of their clients
to perform their health care responsibilities competently. The clarity, time-
liness, and sensitivity of human communication in health care is often critical
to the physical and emotional well-being of all concerned. In compiling a
client's case history the practitioner must be able to evoke clear, accurate,
and detailed information in order to diagnose the current state of health,
identify relevant health experiences, and develop effective strategies for
health care intervention and maintenance.

Regardless of the health care professional's level of scientific expertise,
if he or she does not communicate effectively in establishing the client's
history there will be insufficient information available to direct treatment.
In the course of health care treatment the practitioner must utilize communication skills to gather information from the client, answer the client's
questions, give the client directions for self-care and establish a therapeutic
relationship.

Communication is also pragmatically important and can save the health
care provider from malpractice suits. In order to avoid malpractice, several

insurance companies provide risk management for their clients. The purpose of risk management is to educate health care providers so that they will avoid being sued. Guidelines to avoid law suits include the following points which involve effective communication:

1. Clearly and accurately document what you do and say to clients.
2. Obtain careful informed consent.
3. Have open communication between doctor and clients, doctor and nurses, and among physicians.
4. Pay attention to the balance of clients' rights versus doctor responsibilities.
5. Diffuse client anger. Simple acts of concern and courtesy will often prevent large lawsuits (Gorney, 1988).

Although a natural ability to communicate effectively with people is certainly advantageous to a health care professional, to function as a "professional" demands a more disciplined awareness of the manner in which human interaction occurs. The practitioner needs to develop increased awareness of both the impact of his or her own communication behaviors and the behaviors of others. The competent health care practitioner should be aware of the wide range of verbal and nonverbal messages clients and co-workers transmit in health care situations. For example, in the case history at the beginning of this chapter, if the dentists and the dental assistants had been aware that their client was showing nonverbal cues of discomfort, they could have helped dispel her fears. Because these health care professionals were not alert to their client's communication, they failed to react appropriately and actually aggravated her anxiety. Interpersonal concerns of health care are reviewed in chapter 3.

Effective human communication skills and competencies do not just happen; people are not born with effective communication skills, nor do these competencies necessarily develop naturally. Skills and competencies are learned behaviors that have to be examined and practiced in order to be mastered. This book is designed to direct your examination, practice, and mastery of effective human communication to be used in the delivery of health care services.

Health care relationships are primary channels for acquiring and seeking health information. As such, they are crucial delivery vehicles for a wide range of health care services (Kreps and Thornton, 1984). The communication relationships established by health care providers and consumers have a major influence on the behaviors they engage in during health care practice (Smith, 1976). An unspoken "implicit contract" is developed between relational partners; health care provider/consumer relationships direct interactants to behave in accordance with the behavioral boundaries of each other's role expectations (Kreps, 1986a; Rossiter & Pearce, 1975). The messages they exchange indicate the kinds of roles they expect each other to perform. Effective health care relationships have clearly understood and agreed-upon implicit contracts. Relational partners work at continually updating their awareness of mutual expectations by giving and seeking interpersonal feedback, enabling the partners to continue to act appropriately toward each other as their relationship grows (Kreps, 1986a). Effective health care relationships have major influences on the success of health care, influencing both the outcomes and satisfaction people derive from such situations (Korsch & Negrete, 1972; Lane, 1983, Street & Wiemann, 1987).

The need for knowledge and skills in human communication for health care delivery is not limited just to the physician; all who work in health care benefit from such skills. Members of the health care team must work interdependently with other team members as well as with clients in accomplishing health care tasks. Each individual performs an integral role in the complex and multi-faceted health care delivery system. Teams and groups will be discussed more fully in chapter 4.

The health care delivery system is like a wagon wheel with many different spokes (see Figure 1.1). The hub of the wheel is the client's role. The entire health care system should revolve around the health care needs of consumers. Each of the spokes of the wheel represents one of the health care professional roles. Each of these roles performs important functions for the consumer in the delivery of health care. The client is the point where each of these professional roles meet. The combination of the specific health care skills of each of these professional areas provides the client with health care services. The quality of treatment provided to the client often depends on the effectiveness of human communication between the different parts of the health care delivery wheel.

Active and accurate communication between interdependent health care professionals, as well as between clients and practitioners, enables coordination within the health care system. A breakdown in communication between any of the spokes of the wheel or between any spoke and the hub of the wheel can jeopardize the effectiveness of the entire health care system by weakening the strength of the wheel. Together, all parts of the wheel add strength to the health care system. Effective communication keeps the parts of the health care delivery system working in concert and enhances the quality of health care. Organizational communication will be the focus of chapter 5.

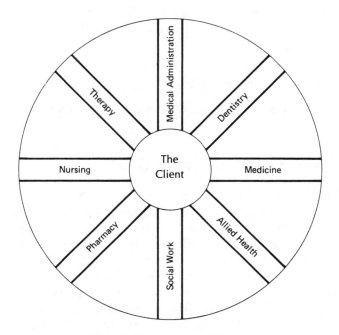

Figure 1.1   The Health-Care Delivery System Wheel.

Problems and Issues in the Delivery of Health Care

Practitioners are often unaware of the ways in which their messages may frighten or confuse clients. Clients often fail to recognize how important it is for them to explain their symptoms clearly and fully to their health care providers in order to receive appropriate treatment. Both clients and practitioners report frustration and dissatisfaction in their health care encounters with others. Korsch and Negrete concluded, in their 1972 *Scientific American* article, "The quality of medical care depends in the last analysis on the interaction of the patient and the doctor, and there is abundant evidence that in current practice this interaction all too often is disappointing to both parties." While more emphasis has been placed on researching communication in health care since that article was written, there is little evidence to indicate that health care communication is much improved.

Kreps (1988) lists five problem areas in health care linked to communication inadequacies:

1. Low levels of patient compliance/cooperation
2. Miscommunication and misinformation
3. Unrealistic and unfulfilled patient expectations linked to cultural stereotypes
4. Insensitivity
5. Dissatisfaction with health care by both providers and consumers

These problem areas will be discussed in the remaining sections of this chapter.

Client Cooperation with Health Care

Poor compliance with prescribed health care programs is often identified as a problem area in health care. The compliance literature addresses such issues as clients' failure to (1) comply with keeping health care appointments, (2) follow health care regimens, (3) use prescribed drugs correctly, or (4) abide by the rules of the health care institution (Lane, 1983).

Compliance is commonly examined in health care research, but it has rarely been studied from a relational communication perspective (Arntson, 1985; Lane, 1983). The primary areas of compliance research have focused on patient compliance with health care appointments (Alpert, 1964; Hertz & Stamps, 1977), regimens (Caron, 1968; Davis & Eichorn, 1963; Lane, 1982), and use of prescribed drugs (Blackwell, 1973; Hulka, Cassel & Kupper, 1976; Hulka, Kupper & Cassell, 1975). Although most of the compliance literature focuses on the characteristics of patients that lead to poor compliance, an interactive perspective on the compliance issue explores the level of cooperation elicited in the provider/consumer relationship (Kreps, 1986d; Kreps & Thornton, 1984; Lane, 1982, 1983). From a relational perspective, the responsibility for health care cooperation is shared jointly by consumer and provider (Arntson, 1985; Speedling & Rose, 1985; Kreps, 1986; Kasl, 1975). Evidence suggests that the quality of interaction between health care providers and consumers strongly influences the level of cooperation between these health communicators (Lane, 1982; Stone, 1979). Low levels of patient compliance have also been linked to the failure to establish effective provider/patient communication relationships (Charney, 1972; Dimatteo, 1979; Lane, 1983, 1982; Stone, 1979). Poor consumer compliance in health care is generally recognized as a major problem impeding the delivery of high-quality health care services.

The identification of this problem area as "patient compliance" indicates a one-way practitioner orientation. The responsibility for poor "compliance" is directed toward the client. In this book, we prefer to speak about compliance in terms of cooperation between the client and the practitioner, where responsibility for health care outcomes are shared jointly by the client and the practitioner.

Cooperation is not a naturally occurring part of human endeavor but rather the outcome of relationship development. Instead of viewing client noncompliance as a maladaptive client characteristic, it is more productive to view the problem as related to the kind of communication relationship established between the client and the practitioner. Health care providers can evoke client cooperation with their medical regimens, directions, appointments, and procedures through the development of effective communication relationships. In chapter 2, we will discuss the relationship development process and suggest strategies for developing effective client-practitioner communication relationships.

Miscommunication in Health Care

Another pervasive problem in the delivery of health care is the misinterpretation of communication between people. This is known as *miscommunication*. Miscommunication does not mean that communication has not occurred. *It means that often the meanings that communicators create in response to messages sent to them are very different from the meanings that were intended.*

Miscommunication occurs in many interpersonal communication situations, often because of the idiosyncratic ways individuals process information. The complexity of health care problems, diagnoses, and treatments makes it difficult to create and interpret health care messages without ambiguities and information loss. The overuse of medical jargon by health care providers often confuses consumers of health care, leading consumers to misinterpret messages (Barnlund, 1976). Miscommunications often cause serious difficulties in health care because they misdirect intricate interdependent health preserving behaviors. They also lead consumers to interpret incorrectly the health care instructions explained to them by providers, making it virtually impossible to comply with health care regimens. Providers, on their side, can misinterpret messages patients give them, resulting in incorrect diagnoses and in inappropriate treatments. Health care providers and consumers must communicate clearly and seek feedback to avoid miscommunications (Cline, 1983; Kreps & Thornton, 1984).

Miscommunication is not indigenous solely to health care interaction. It occurs regularly between people in all kinds of social, business and educational situations. The reason miscommunication in health care is of such vital importance is the crucial need for accurate and timely information regarding client diagnosis and treatment. Sometimes it can literally be a matter of life or death. For example, if a hospital lab technician reports the results of a client's blood test to the client's attending physician over the telephone (as sometimes is the case in busy hospitals), there is a good opportunity for miscommunication to occur. An inaccuracy of even one decimal point in reporting these blood test results can strongly affect the physician's diagnosis of the client and the regimen prescribed. An incorrect diagnosis and prescription would undoubtedly complicate the original health problem, with the ultimate potential of endangering the client's life.

Misunderstandings between clients and their health care providers can be a cause of noncompliance. It is difficult for a client to follow a health care regimen that he or she does not understand. Part of establishing an effective practitioner-client relationship is being able to communicate clearly, honestly, and accurately. In chapter 2 we will discuss the use of verbal and nonverbal messages in communicating meaningfully with others, as well as the utilization of feedback in human communication to counteract the problem of miscommunication.

Unrealistic Expectations in Health Care

Another source of problems in the delivery of health care arises from unrealistic expectations held by both clients and professionals concerning each other's performance and the outcomes of health care treatment. Studies have indicated that health care professionals and clients tend to stereotype one another. These stereotypes are often unrealistic generalizations of the attitudes, inclinations, and abilities of people in health care situations (Davis, 1971, 1968).

Unrealistic and unfulfilled expectations have been linked to cultural stereotypes, misinterpretations of relational needs, and inflexible relational role performances (Blackwell, 1973; Fuller & Queseda, 1973; Mechanic, 1972; Myerhoff & Larson, 1965; Walker, 1973). Often stereotyping, misinformation and inflexibility are caused by unconscious, nonverbal cultural cues and information.

Consumers may enter the health care situation expecting the health care professional to perform minor miracles — eradicating their ailments and making them better than they were before. The doctor is often seen as a cultural hero by the public, able to solve any and all problems. Doctors on the TV series "General Hospital" may be able to solve all of their clients' problems, but it is impossible for real-life doctors to do the same. These unrealistic stereotypes put the health care professional in an untenable position — they can never meet clients' expectations.

Health care professionals also stereotype their clients. Research has indicated that health care professionals prefer certain clients over others. Depending on age, illness-type, sex, status, or level of attractiveness, a client may be stereotyped in different ways by the health care professional. Different stereotypes receive differing styles of treatment. Health care providers also often underestimate their clients' level of understanding of their health care treatments and problems. These unrealistic evaluations of clients can inhibit high quality health care delivery.

Lack of Sensitivity in Health Care

Insensitive communication between health care providers and their clients is also an issue. Insensitivity may be the greatest source of dissatisfaction people feel about the health care system. Due to heavy workloads, high stress, and constant contact with human suffering, the health care professional may become callous to the feelings of others. Practitioners can become "burnt-out" after extended tours of duty on busy hospital wards, making them less responsive to the needs of their clients.

Clients also have been known to be insensitive toward the needs and feelings of their providers. They often see their own problems as preeminent over the problems of others. The consumer may demand immediate attention and become belligerent when the practitioner cannot instantly leave whatever he or she is doing and respond to the client. Certainly, upon reflection, the client's sense of urgency is understandable. Clients can become apprehensive and fearful about their health condition; because of their fear they can see only their own problems. Insensitivity in health care has been related to low levels of interpersonal respect, attempts for relational control, and inability to interpret nonverbal messages accurately (Kane & Deuschle, 1967; Korsch, Gozzi & Francis, 1968; Korsch and Negrete, 1972; Lane, 1982).

We certainly do not intend to imply that all health care practitioners and consumers practice insensitive communication. There are many extremely sensitive individuals in health care. Yet, the people who do behave in an unfeeling way to others can cause health care problems. The previous health care problems we have identified (cooperation, miscommunication, and unrealistic expectations) are strongly related to insensitive communication.

Dissatisfaction with Health Care Services

Health care problems such as those we have just discussed have caused widespread dissatisfaction. One serious consequence of dissatisfaction is that people who need health care treatment may avoid seeking professional help. Clients who receive health care services are not always satisfied with their treatment, which may relate to the increase in health care malpractice suits. Health care professionals who are dissatisfied with their roles and outcomes in health care practice are more likely to become disenchanted with the health care system, eventually leading to burnout and turnover of health care staff.

Dissatisfaction with health care by both providers and consumers has been tied to failure to express interpersonal empathy, relational equality, and caring (Kane & Deuschle, 1967; Korsch, Gozzi & Francis, 1968; Korsch & Negrete, 1972; Lane, 1983; Street & Wiemann, 1987).

Political, Legal, and Ethical Aspects of the Health Care System

Communication does not take place in a vacuum and health care providers and consumers are strongly influenced by the system in which health care takes place. Different countries as well as different parts of the same country sometimes do not have the same philosophy toward illness or toward the political, legal and ethical aspects of health care (Payer, 1988). Organizational, political, and system issues will be discussed in chapter 5; culture and ethics will be addressed in chapters 7 and 8.

As health care is expected to consume from 12 to 13 percent of the gross national product at the turn of the century, the legal and economic issues are of increasing concern. These issues in turn affect the communication process. For example, the increasing tendency of consumers to sue their physicians is one of the reasons for the many tests given to a client before surgery. Requiring these tests when they are not needed by the consumer raises many economic, legal and ethical issues.

Summary

Human communication is strongly related to each of the health care problem areas we have identified. We have linked client cooperation to the establishment of effective communication relationships. Miscommunications are caused by ineffective use of messages and feedback in health care. Unrealistic expectations of health care are based on over-generalized perceptions and stereotypes of the people involved in the health care system. Lack of sensitivity in health care causes people to communicate callously with one another, and precipitates the breakdown of health care relationships. All of these problems lead to dissatisfaction with health care and loss of effectiveness in the health care delivery system. Improvement in human communication in health care will certainly not solve all of the problems that are part of the complex health care system, but it can help improve the levels of satisfaction people have with their health care relationships.

CHAPTER

2

Health Communication Processes and Theories

Rhonda and David Coleman had been married for nine years but had not been able to have the children they very much wanted. When a new obstetrician-gynecologist moved to their area they were delighted to hear that he was a fertility expert. They began treatment with Dr. Dolan. After six months, Rhonda became pregnant. The couple was elated and chose to continue with Dr. Dolan. Rhonda did have some reservations about this decision as she had found communication with him difficult, but his obvious technical and medical skills attracted both of the Colemans.

The Colemans' joy about the pregnancy turned into a nightmare during the following nine months. Rhonda was apprehensive because of her history. Dr. Dolan was brusque and noncommunicative when he was examining her, and the examinations were efficient but brief. Appearing overworked and exasperated, he even suggested one time that she go to the local bookstore and buy some books on pregnancy that would make her a more informed patient so that she wouldn't have so many questions. Rhonda came home in tears, but the couple was afraid to change doctors at that point in the pregnancy.

Rhonda called a friend who was a nurse. She was helpful in answering many questions and alleviating some of Rhonda and David's concerns. At the end of nine months Rhonda went into labor. The long labor was difficult partly because of her uneasiness with and distrust of Dr. Dolan.

After giving birth to a healthy baby, the Colemans found Dr. Allard, a pediatrician whom they liked and admired. One of their criteria at that point was communication, and the pediatrician they chose took time to reassure families and answer questions. When the Colemans told of their ordeal with the obstetrician-gynecologist, Dr. Allard agreed to talk to Dr. Dolan, who was a friend as well as a colleague. Dr. Dolan was terribly distressed at hearing the Colemans' complaints. He had assumed they were simply grateful to have a healthy baby. After further talks, Dr. Dolan admitted that he had had other complaints about his ability to communicate. He finally agreed that he must do something about this problem. What should he do? How could he learn to understand and improve his communication?

The Nature of Human Communication

Perhaps the greatest problem with human communication in health care is the assumption that communication is an easy thing to do well. This assumption is only half true. It is easy to communicate, but it is difficult to communicate well. Even though we have been communicating with others all of our lives, we are not always effective communicators. In this chapter, we will discuss the nature of human communication, examine the major aspects of the communication process, and identify strategies for communicating effectively in health care.

Human communication occurs when a person responds to a message and assigns meaning to it. The two key parts to this definition of human communication are the *message* and the *meaning*. Messages are anything that people attend to and create meanings for in the communication process. Messages can take many different forms. They can be spoken words, written words, facial expressions, environmental cues, temperatures, thoughts, or feelings. Basically, there are two groups of messages: *internal messages*, those we send to ourselves, and *external messages*, those we react to from our environment (including other people). Meanings are mental images we create to develop a sense of understanding. People respond to messages (emanating both internally and externally) and create meanings for these messages when communicating.

Human communication occurs at various levels. The most basic level of human communication is *intrapersonal communication*. Intrapersonal communication occurs when we communicate with ourselves. People constantly have an ongoing internal dialogue of thoughts. For example, health care practitioners constantly use intrapersonal communication to make choices about client care, to interpret messages from clients and co-workers, and to decide how to explain health concepts and treatments to their clients. The intrapersonal process for creating messages is known as *encoding*, and the intrapersonal process of interpreting messages is known as *decoding*.

Both encoding and decoding are translation processes people use to link the two most crucial elements of communication together: meanings and messages. In the encoding process, the health practitioner translates the meanings he or she has about a given situation into the most appropriate messages available for use in communicating with others. Decoding is the translation of messages into meanings. Intrapersonal communication is the most basic form of human communication because the processes of encoding and decoding enable people to send and receive messages, which in turn make it possible for them to communicate on interpersonal, small group, and organizational levels.

Interpersonal communication is communication between two people (a dyad), usually face-to-face, although people can use communication media (such as the telephone) to communicate interpersonally without being in each other's immediate presence. Interpersonal communication builds upon intrapersonal communication because each member of the interpersonal dyad must communicate with him or her self to communicate effectively with each other. Intrapersonal and interpersonal levels of communication occur simultaneously when one person speaks with another person. The interpersonal communicator uses intrapersonal communication to decode the messages of the other person with whom he or she is communicating and to encode messages he or she intends to send to the other person.

One of the most important outcomes of interpersonal communication is the development of human relationships. As we discussed in the first chapter, people depend on their interpersonal relationships to elicit cooperation from others. In chapter 3, we will detail the importance of establishing effective client-practitioner relationships in the delivery of health care. As with intrapersonal communication, the interpersonal level of communication facilitates communication at the next higher level of human communication — the small group.

Small group communication occurs when three or more people interact with one another in an attempt to adapt to their environment and achieve commonly recognized goals. As in interpersonal communication, small group communication usually occurs face-to-face but may also develop through use of communication media (for example, teleconferencing). The total number of small group communicators is generally limited to the number of people who can actively participate in a group conversation.

Small group communication is more complex than interpersonal communication because group interaction is composed of many different interpersonal communication relationships. As the number of communicators within the small group increases, the complexity of the communication situation increases geometrically due to the number of potential message exchanges that can occur between group members. For example, Bostrom (1970) has calculated that a group of eight people has a possibility of 1,056 interactions.

Another aspect of group communication that differs from interpersonal communication is the dimension of *group dynamics*. Group dynamics is the potential for the development of subgroups and opposing coalitions within the group membership. The development of these coalitions complicates group communication and the relationships between group members. The different ways group dynamics can develop within a group can have a strong impact on the output of the group.

The small group is an important work unit in health care. Small group communication occurs in health care teams, therapy groups, consumer education classes, and decision-making committees within health care organizations. These groups perform important functions in the health care system by providing information, support, and problem solving abilities that individuals couldn't possibly provide independently. In chapter 4, we will explore the functions and processes of small group communication in health care, emphasizing the development and operation of effective health care teams.

The fourth and most complex level of human communication is *organizational communication*. An organization is a social system composed of interdependent groups of people working toward commonly recognized goals. Organizational communication refers to human communication between organization members during the performance of their organizational tasks. Organizational communication encompasses all the prior levels of communication — intrapersonal, interpersonal, and small group.

Organizational communication is integral to the functioning of health care institutions because it is the means by which health care practitioners (from all aspects of the health care system) coordinate their activities to accomplish the goals of the organization. Because of the great size and complexity of many modern health care organizations it is virtually impossible to have face-to-face communication between all members of the organization. To cope with the complexity of organizational communication, formal channels of communication between different parts and members of the organization must be established. We will discuss in much greater depth some current communication problems and coping mechanisms for health care organizations in chapter 7.

In summary, there are four levels of human communication that build upon one another and increase in complexity from intrapersonal communication to interpersonal communication to small group communication to organizational communication. Figure 2.1 illustrates the hierarchical nature of the four basic levels of human communication.

As you can see in Figure 2.1, intrapersonal communication is the largest and most basic form of human communication. It is at the intrapersonal level that we think and process information. Interpersonal communication builds upon the intrapersonal level, adding another person to the communication situation and introducing the dyadic relationship. Small group communication, in turn, builds upon interpersonal interaction, utilizing several

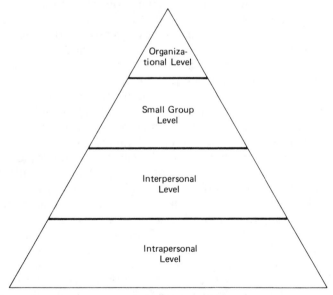

Figure 2.1   Hierarchical Levels of Human Communication

communicators and adding the new dimensions of group dynamics and multiple interpersonal relationships to the communication situation. Organizational communication exists through the combination of the three previous levels of communication in coordinating large numbers of people in the shared accomplishment of complex goals. It is important to recognize how each of the higher levels of communication is dependent upon the effectiveness of its lower levels of communication. Effective communication at each level is developed through effective communication at preceding levels.

In addition to these four basic levels of human communication, there are also two special forms of communication that do not fit neatly into our hierarchy but utilize elements from each of the levels: *public communication* and *mass communication*. Public communication occurs when a small number of people (usually only one person) addresses a larger group of people. Although the speaker takes the major responsibility for the public communication and sends the preponderance of verbal messages, that person is not the only person engaging in communication. The audience also sends messages to the speaker, primarily through nonverbal channels. Speeches, lectures, oral reports, and dramatic performances are all forms of public communication.

Mass communication occurs when a small number of people send messages to a large, anonymous, and usually heterogeneous audience through the use of some specialized communication medium. Mass communication uses such diverse media as film, television, radio, newspapers, books, and magazines. Mass communication is similar to public communication in that the person delivering the message takes primary responsibility for the communication. However, mass communication has the potential for reaching larger audiences than face-to-face public communication, and has less opportunity for audience participation.

Both public communication and mass communication have the advantage of being able to reach large audiences, thereby communicating with many people in a short amount of time. On the other hand, both forms of communication also have the disadvantage of limited shared communication with the audience. The reactions of an audience to communication is known as *feedback*. As we will discuss later in this chapter, feedback plays an important part of communication by both clarifying and humanizing human interaction. To maximize the advantages of public and mass communication while minimizing their disadvantages, an effective communicator employs intrapersonal, interpersonal, small group, and organizational levels of communication. By using all of these forms of communication, the health care provider can reach a large number of people in a clear and personal manner. Throughout the rest of this book, we will examine the ways in which health care professionals can utilize all of these levels of human communication.

Communication as Process

Human communication is a *dynamic, ongoing process — communication does not start and stop.* People are constantly involved in communicating with themselves and with other people. We are immersed in a sea of messages and meanings. *Human beings cannot not communicate.* As long as you are alive, you are involved in some form of communication.

It is easy to oversimplify the human communication process. Many early models of human communication assumed that one person (a source, or sender) sent a message to another person (a receiver) in communication. This is an oversimplification. No one individual is only a sender or a receiver in human communication. *In human communication we simultaneously send and receive many messages on many different levels.* We are constantly encoding and decoding. These early linear models of human communication fail to recognize the continuously developing nature of the communication phenomenon.

By seeing communication as an ongoing process you must recognize that human *communication is irreversible.* Human *communication is bound to the context in which it occurs.* Context refers to the time and space surrounding human communication. When communication occurs and how people feel about the timing of the communication has a major impact. For example, it is a far different communication situation depending on whether a friend phones you at 8 P.M. or at 3 A.M.! Time also refers to the day of the week and month of the year, and so forth. The setting where communication occurs also has great impact on the interaction. You certainly communicate differently with people in a class, at a party, in a clinic, or on a hospital ward. Even if you say exactly the same thing in several different situations to the same people, the changes in context will inevitably alter the communication that takes place.

Once you have communicated something to someone, you cannot retract it. The communication event that transpired became permanent the moment it occurred. By restating or changing the messages sent you do not remove previous messages, you merely add on to them. For example, a nurse tells a hospitalized client to prepare for surgery and later finds out the client is not scheduled for surgery until the next day. No matter how many times the nurse explains the mistake, the impact of the communication on the client remains. It is similar to a judge in a courtroom murder trial telling the jury to disregard an outburst from a courtroom spectator who yells that the defendant is a killer. No matter how the judge implores the jury to be impartial, the communication has had its effect. The irreversible nature of human communication underscores the importance of careful communication in health care. Whatever the health care professional says, it will always be remembered to some extent.

Human communication is a deceptively complex process. There are many different aspects of communication that interrelate in the communication phenomenon. In this book we will take a *transactional* perspective on human communication. Transactionality implies that communication is a process composed of myriad components interacting simultaneously to produce communication. Some of these key components include the messages to which people react, the meanings people actively create, the time and place of the communication (context), the relationships established between communicators, the past experiences of the communicators, the personalities and dispositions of the communicators, the purposes people have for communicating, and the effects of human communication on people and situations. Throughout this book we will be examining communication in health care from a transactional perspective, identifying the crucial parts of the communication process and determining the effects of human communication on the delivery of health care services.

Communication and the Creation of Meaning

Human beings have an insatiable appetite for creating meanings. We strive to know what is going on around us, to understand the people with whom we interact, and to get a handle on the different situations in which we find ourselves. Human communication is the primary tool we use to develop a sense of understanding people and situations. We gather information from the messages available to us and interpret these messages to create satisfying meanings to help us cope effectively with the world around us.

The creation of meaning is a very personal process. *All people are unique and their perceptions of reality and creations of meaning are unique.* We have the cognitive ability to create very rich, deep meanings at many different levels. Because the creation of meaning is a personal process, we each create unique meanings often interpreting the same situation in very different ways. The creation of meaning is not a mechanical process; it is part of a learned psychological process.

Meanings are in people, not in words, objects, or things. People actively create meanings in response to the world around them. No object or word has inherent meaning. Human beings create meanings for words and objects in order to understand this complex universe.

Selective Perception

Human perception is a process by which people become aware of internal and external messages and interpret these messages into meanings. Human beings perceive the world around them through the use of their sensory mechanisms. These sensory mechanisms include sight, hearing, touch, taste, smell, balance, awareness of heat, cold, pain, pleasure, and pressure. In addition to perceiving *external messages* through use of our senses, we also perceive internally generated messages. *Internal messages* are both physiologically oriented (as in feelings of hunger, fatigue, or nervousness) and mentally oriented (as in thinking, daydreaming, and choice making).

An important internal channel of mentally oriented messages is something we label "channel Z" or the ability to imagine and create rich fantasies. Channel Z is a mental mechanism people create to transport themselves from their physical environment to a convivial fantasy land of their own making. Humans' ability to enter channel Z can be very therapeutic for them if they use their imaginations in appropriate situations. Use of channel Z can be a refreshing and rejuvenating experience, helping people cope with stressful situations by providing them with an important repose from reality. Some people are unable to control their use of channel Z, daydreaming and fantasizing in inappropriate situations when they should be focusing their attention on externally generated messages. The ability to control perceptual processes is an important communication skill.

A major problem in controlling human perception is the overwhelming number of potential messages available to the perceiver. People cannot possibly perceive everything there is in any given situation, even if they are able to block out their own internally generated messages, because of the extensive range of external messages. People have a limited amount of *cognitive space* for processing information. If we attempted to perceive all of the messages available to us, we would suffer from *information overload*. The overload resulting from our inability to process all of the messages bombarding us would leave us disoriented and confused.

To complicate the perceptual process even more, people don't have the ability to perceive everything around them due to their *sensory limitations*. There are limitations on our hearing, sight, smell, and so on. We cannot hear all of the sounds around us or see all of the light waves bombarding us.

Human beings have developed the cognitive process of *selective perception* to maximize the effectiveness of the messages they do perceive and minimize the perceptual problems caused by cognitive and sensory limitations. Selective perception is a process by which people select the most important messages out of the total pool of potentially perceivable messages and use those selected messages to make sense out of their current situation. There are three interrelated parts to the selective perception process. They are:

1. *Selective Attention*: focusing on the key messages in any situation;
2. *Habituation*: eliminating extraneous or unimportant messages in any situation;
3. *Closure*: putting together the messages collected through selective attention and arranging them into a meaningful configuration.

The messages people select through selective attention are chosen due to the unique past experiences and predispositions of each individual. Not only do people select the most important messages around them through selective attention, but they also prioritize these messages. The most important messages are given the most cognitive space (attention), and the less important messages are afforded less cognitive space. Every split second, people update the selective attention choices they have made and reprioritize the messages they have selected.

Selective attention and habituation work hand in hand and operate simultaneously. In order to give full attention to any set of messages, an individual must be able to block out competing messages. This is why habituation is so important. To habituate effectively, people must be able to block out both external messages and internal messages. External messages that compete for attention might be noises or distracting visual cues while competing internal messages might be fatigue or daydreams. People develop their ability to habituate well through continued practice.

The individual must then provide closure: make sense out of the situation based on limited information gathered from the messages which were received. This is done by filling in the blank spaces between messages through educated assumptions based on the perceiver's past experiences and sense of logic. The better individuals are at creating closure, the more likely they are to develop a strong sense of understanding for the perceptual situation.

Since each person develops his or her own method of perceiving the world through individualized versions of selective perception, it is likely that different people will select different messages on which to focus. Additionally, they will block out different messages and put the messages they have attended to together in different ways. These individual differences in the selective perception process are the primary reasons for divergent creations of meaning. There is no objective reality, only subjective realities created by different people based on individual perceptions of the world. The major implication derived from perceptual differences between people is the need for interpersonal communication to check and clarify the meanings people create. *People cannot exchange meanings: they can exchange messages.* The more effective the messages they send to one another, the more likely it is that communicators will be able to create overlapping (similar) meanings, thereby developing communicative understanding for one another.

Content and Relationship Levels of Communication

Messages people send one another have both a *content* and *relationship* dimension. The content aspect of human communication refers to the basic, tangible information being presented in the message. The primary topic, theme, and data of what is being said is contained within the content level of communication. The relationship level of communication, on the other hand, refers to the feelings communicators express for each other through their communication. Expressions of respect/disrespect, like/dislike, powerfulness/powerlessness, love/hate, or comfort/discomfort are all parts of the relationship dimension of human communication. The content and relationship aspects of human communication are expressed simultaneously in every message sent and received in interpersonal communication. Since interpersonal communicators send and receive a multitude of messages all the time, content and relationship levels of messages have a major impact on interpersonal communication. It is important to recognize that every time you tell someone something you are not merely expressing information about the topic but you are also defining the relationship you are in the process of establishing with your communication partner.

Even the most common statement (for example, "How's it going?") has content and relationship communication aspects. On a content level the statement expresses an inquiry into the status of the receiver's mental, physical, and social condition at that given moment, as well as expressing a greeting from one person to another. On a relationship level the statement might imply concern for the receiver's well-being, interpersonal attraction between the sender and the receiver of the message, empathy for the receiver's current situation, or merely an expression of friendship.

The content level of communication provides people with information about the world around them. As we discussed earlier in this chapter, people have an insatiable appetite for knowing about the environment in which they live and the people to whom they relate. The world is a complex and confusing place. Information helps people understand the world around them by reducing the uncertainty they have about other people and things.

Every situation has a certain level of uncertainty. We never know everything there is to know about any given person, place, or situation. Every bit of information we gather through content communication provides us with more knowledge about the world around us. The content level of human communication helps us to understand the world we live in and to cope with uncertainty.

The relationship level of human communication provides people with information about the relationships they are developing with others. We are in constant need of human companionship. Human beings are social creatures and depend on their relationships with others to provide mutual emotional support to solve difficult problems and to coordinate complex activities.

Every time a message is sent between people, at least one aspect of that message communicates something about the relationship. Relationships are established and develop through communication. Every time you communicate with someone, you are affecting your relationship with that person in some way. Communication can increase or break down the effectiveness of human relationships, depending on the relative degree of personal or object communication inherent in the messages being communicated.

The relationship aspect of interpersonal messages can be placed on a continuum between *personal and object communication*. Personal communication shows respect for the other person. A communicator sending messages on the personal end of the continuum (see Figure 2.2) communicates with the other person as an equal, allows the other person's perspective to affect the messages sent, and generally communicates in an honest and trustworthy manner. Object communication, on the other hand, is insensitive and demonstrates lack of respect for the other person. It tells the person what to do without seeking his or her input on the matter and treats the other person as an unintelligent and unimportant being.

Personal communication tends to be a humanizing form of human interaction, while object communication tends to be a dehumanizing form of human interaction as Figure 2.2 illustrates. Personal communication makes us feel good about ourselves. It bolsters our self-image by communicating the relational message that who we are and what we have to say is important. Conversely, object communication tears down our self-image; it makes us question our worth, and we become angry at the person treating us as an object rather than as a person.

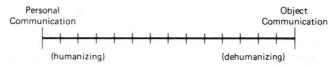

Figure 2.2   Continuum of Personal and Object Communication

Since personal and object communication are parts of the relational aspect of communication, it is possible to communicate the same general content information in very different relational ways using either personal or object level messages. For example, a dentist can ask a client to cooperate with a dental regimen in either a personal or object manner. On the object level, "If you don't brush your teeth regularly it won't be much longer until you have no teeth," or on a more personal level, "If you'd consider brushing your teeth every day, you will counteract the buildup of tooth decay and make your teeth last longer." The object approach to client communication treats the client as though he or she had to be bullied into complying with the dental regimen, while the personal approach treats the client as a responsible individual who will cooperate with the dentist if given good reasons. Which manner of communication would you prefer?

Personal communication can be beneficial to the establishment of effective client-practitioner relationships. Object communication, on the other hand, can be detrimental to effective client-practitioner relationships. It takes no more time to communicate personally with people than it does to communicate in an object manner. It does take respect, honesty, and a genuine concern for yourself and the other person. Throughout the rest of the book we will consider the perils of communicating on an object level. We will also explore strategies for utilizing personal communication in client-practitioner relationships, health care teams, health care organizations, and in developing therapeutic communication.

Communication and Feedback

As we discussed earlier in this chapter, *feedback* is a communicated response to another individual's communication. It functions by providing communicators with information about how they are being perceived by others. With this feedback, communicators can adjust their message strategies to communicate more effectively. Because feedback guides people in adjusting the messages they send to one another, it helps to clarify human communication.

Effective communicators constantly seek feedback from the people with whom they are communicating to determine how these people are reacting to the communication situation. Intrapersonally, you send yourself feedback about your thoughts or actions when you review your ideas and behaviors. Interpersonally, feedback helps you determine what effects your communications are having upon your dyadic partners and how they feel about you. In small groups feedback is used to determine the ideas and reactions of group members about problems and their solutions. In organizations, feedback determines the adequacy of member information and effectiveness of organizational policies. In public communication, feedback allows the speaker to gauge the responses of the audience to his or her presentation. Even in mass communication, where feedback works most slowly, feedback is needed to evaluate the effectiveness of a mass communicated event or program.

Seeking feedback from people in communication situations is a way of humanizing the interpersonal interaction. It is important for health care providers not only because it gives them information about the level of information the client possesses, but also because it communicates to the client that the health care professional is interested in his or her perspective on the health care situation.

Metacommunication is a specialized form of feedback about the manner in which people communicate. Metacommunication is communication about communication; the communicator is given feedback about the way he or she is communicating. *Metacommunication is a primary tool in socialization because rules of interaction are learned from metacommunicative processes.*

Every human relationship, group, organization, and culture develops rules for the ways in which people are supposed to communicate. Later on in this book, we will discuss these communication rules in more depth, identifying them as norms. Some of these rules include the accepted manner of address people have for one another, the type of dress codes that exist, the use of specialized language (jargon, slang, or foreign languages), and the ways in which people are allowed to touch each other in different situations. The primary function of metacommunication is to teach people the correct rules for communicating.

When you were a child, you were probably given many metacommunication messages to teach you how to act correctly in different situations. For example, children are often taught how to speak politely with metacommunicative messages like, "Always say thank you when you are given a present, even if you don't like the present." As people grow older, the metacommunicative messages they receive become more subtle. Usually adults teach other adults communication rules by using less obvious nonverbal metacommunicative messages. When a person breaks a communication rule, his or her contemporaries will usually indicate nonverbally through a frown, a harsh look, or laughter that what that person has said or done is not acceptable.

Some people are less perceptive about metacommunicative messages than others. These people are often shunned by others because they don't act in accordance with social rules. To be effective in any communication situation, whether it be interpersonal, group, or organizational, you must be able to recognize metacommunication messages and learn the rules for appropriate communication behaviors. We will discuss metacommunication again in relation to learning group and cultural norms.

Verbal and Nonverbal Message Systems

Messages are the tools people use to communicate with one another. As we discussed earlier in this chapter, people exchange messages to evoke each other's creation of meaning. We identified two kinds of messages: internally generated messages (thoughts) and externally generated messages. Human beings use these external messages to communicate with one another. There are two kinds of external messages, verbal and nonverbal.

Verbal message systems include the use of words and language, both spoken and written, while *nonverbal message systems* include the wide range of messages people perceive and assign meaning to that are in addition to the use of words. Nonverbal communication contains many different kinds of message systems, ranging from body movements to environmental cues.

Verbal and nonverbal communication often work closely together. In fact, there is no way to use verbal communication (words) without using some form of nonverbal communication. Nonverbal messages always surround and influence the verbal messages people send because the medium used for sending verbal messages is always nonverbal (as in vocal or visual cues). Later on in this chapter we will discuss in more depth the relationships between verbal and nonverbal communication.

Verbal communication is a *digital* form of communication — words represent objects or things. Digital communication is based on the use of an arbitrary symbol system designed to name some phenomenon. Words are not the things they name. They are symbols that are used to signify some experience. There is nothing about the words "tree" or "house" that directly describe either a tree or a house. Language is a synthetic means of communication because people designate which word will stand for which experience. This is one of the main reasons we stated earlier in this chapter that meanings are in people, not in the words people use.

Nonverbal communication is generally an *analogic* form of communication, in that nonverbal messages actually describe the phenomenon they are communicating. Analogic communication is based on the use of symbols that have a likeness to the objects they are representing. Nonverbal messages like facial expressions, postures, gestures, or vocal cues directly represent the feelings and emotional states of the communicator expressing them.

There are some significant differences between analogic and digital modes of communication. Analogic communication is primarily used to communicate emotionally-oriented information, while digital communication is used for communicating data-oriented, technical information. To take this one step further, nonverbal communication (primarily analogic) is most effective at conveying relationship information, and verbal communication (primarily digital) is most effective at conveying content information. It is difficult to convey very technical, complex information nonverbally, and it is equally difficult to express an intense emotional feeling to someone with words (unless these words are surrounded by powerful nonverbal messages such as vocal volume, touch, or eye-contact). Watzlawick, Beavin and Jackson (1967) go so far as to write, "Indeed, wherever relationship is the central issue of communication, we find that digital language is almost meaningless."

The implications of the relationships between verbal communication, digital modes, and content information indicate that words are effective at expressing complex technical topics. The relationships between nonverbal communication, analogic modes, and relationship information imply that emotionally charged information is best suited to nonverbal messages, and that nonverbal communication has a strong effect on defining and developing interpersonal relationships.

Language as a transmitter of complex information has performed an important *timebinding* function for humanity. Timebinding is the storing of human knowledge and experiences and the conveying of this knowledge over time. Written language has provided humankind with a relatively permanent, stable, and widespread source of information. The development of computer languages and advanced technologies will allow present and future generations to timebind information and to process complex messages more effectively than ever before.

Verbal communication is usually thought of only in the spoken mode, but written language is also an important part of verbal communication. The spoken word allows people to communicate about information in a personal and dynamic manner. Yet, it is common for people to forget or misinterpret information that was spoken. The spoken word is very transitory, the words fly past us so quickly at times that it may be difficult to understand all of the messages being sent. In written communication, however, you can usually read at your own rate, as well as carefully review difficult parts of the text. The transitory nature of spoken communication underscores the importance of actively using feedback when speaking with others. Written communication, although less dramatic than spoken interaction, has the advantage of stability, permanence, and formality. To derive the benefits of both spoken and written communication, it is wise to use one to augment the other when you want to make an impact on the person with whom you are communicating and when you also want a formal record of your messages.

There are four interrelated perspectives on the study of verbal communication:

1. *Phonemics*: Examination of the performance of spoken language focusing on the sounds and pronunciations of words.
2. *Syntactics*: Examination of the structural aspects of language usage, emphasizing the grammar of verbal communication.
3. *Semantics*: Examination of the meanings associated with words, developing such tools as dictionaries and thesauri.
4. *Pragmatics*: Examination of the behavioral functions of language use by people in different situations.

In this book we will be most concerned with the semantic and pragmatic aspects of language.

As we discussed earlier in this chapter, meaning is a very rich mental process, and the study of semantics recognizes the depth of human meanings for words by separating meanings into two major types, *denotations* and *connotations*. Denotations are the generally accepted public meanings words have assigned to them. Definitions that you might find in a dictionary are the denotative meanings of language. Connotations are more personal, subjective meanings people create and assign to words. While the denotative meanings associated with words are usually limited to less than ten, the connotative meanings any word might evoke are limitless. These many different denotative and connotative meanings assigned to language reinforce the importance of seeking feedback to check a person's perceptions of words and meanings.

The pragmatic perspective in language examines the ways in which language is used in different situations by different people. An important area of pragmatic language use in health care is the use (and sometimes overuse) of *jargon*. Jargon is a secretive linguistic code used by different groups of people. Sometimes jargon is technical in nature, while at other times jargon is used to communicate social information. Jargon serves a variety of functions for its users including:

1. *Expedites interaction* by combining complex concepts and terms into a single word or phrase that can be recognized by other group members. Examples of this expediting function might include use of abbreviations to communicate lengthy health care concepts such as: Ob-Gyn, CPR, or MRI, as well as short terms in place of more complex ones such as coding, prepping, or detox.
2. *Establishes group membership* by identifying individuals with access to specialized vocabulary and information. If you can use the jargon

of a specialized group of people such as occupational therapists, medical administrators, orthodontists, or neurosurgeons, you are far more likely to evoke cooperation from these individuals when speaking to them about their specialized area because you can identify yourself as being knowledgeable about that specific topic. On the other hand, if you use health care jargon incorrectly, you will immediately identify yourself as a novice!

3. *Creates status* for users over nonusers of the specialized linguistic vocabulary. People sometimes use jargon to impress or intimidate the uninitiated by making those who do not understand the jargon feel confused and foolish. In health care, as in all organizational systems, information is powerful. Jargon users can attempt to establish power over nonusers by intimating through their word choices that they possess specialized knowledge and information about health care that the nonusers do not. Establishing power, however, may not be such a good strategy in health care practice because it can cause the relationship to deteriorate and interfere with cooperation between the communicators. Moreover, use of specialized jargon with nonusers will most certainly block the communication of information because the nonusers have no denotative meanings for the jargon terms and phrases. Dr. Kenneth Walker discussed this use of jargon calling it the "me God, you moron" system of communication utilized by many of his physician colleagues. Walker sees this as a way physicians can put themselves on a pedestal and not communicate because they basically do not want to do so (Woods, 1975).

4. *Insulates* users of jargon from nonusers. Jargon use can be used to protect the group of jargon users from infiltration by outside groups of people who do not understand the specialized language. This function of jargon can be useful when a health care professional needs to communicate specialized information that for reasons of confidentiality should not be known by others. The health care provider can use jargon to explain the situation to a peer without risking loss of confidentiality if nongroup members happen to overhear the communication exchange. On the other hand, this insulating aspect of jargon can frustrate others who would like to know what the health care professional is talking about and believe they have a legitimate right to possess the health care information.

As you can see, jargon can be used in many different ways in health care practice. Some of the uses of jargon are extremely beneficial to the health care delivery system, while other uses of jargon may be detrimental to high quality health care. Improper use of jargon in health care can alienate users of jargon from nonusers. The unnecessary use of jargon can be a form of object communication and can cause the nonusers to feel dehumanized. The decision whether or not to use jargon in different health care situations is an ethical decision health care practitioners have to make. In chapter 8, we will discuss the impact of health care ethics on the communication that occurs in health care situations.

Human language is a tool that is used in different ways by different groups of people. Language changes with the needs of people. Because language is constantly changing and evolving to fulfill the needs of its speakers, human language is an emergent phenomenon. To be an effective user of language, you must be able to keep up with the changes and developments in language use. Not only are new words developed and introduced into the language, but existing words also develop new usages. Because information and knowledge are stored and transmitted through language, it is important for language to be in constant flux and development to keep up with our growth in human knowledge. Nowhere has human knowledge expanded more rapidly than in the medical and health care sciences, so it is important for health care professionals to learn current linguistic additions so that they can keep up with this growth in knowledge. This can be done by reading current literature and talking to other professionals.

As indicated earlier in this chapter, nonverbal communication refers to the wide variety of messages people perceive and assign meaning to that are in addition to verbal communication. In essence, this is saying that nonverbal communication is *every possible message source* people respond to besides words. Moreover, as we discussed earlier, nonverbal communication surrounds and influences all verbal communication.

There are many different types of nonverbal messages, and to lump them all together under the extremely general rubric of "nonverbal communication" would be simplistic and confusing. Rather, we will identify seven different, but interrelated, nonverbal systems. These systems work together, usually simultaneously, in human communication. They are:

1. *Artifactics*: People's personal appearances, body shapes, sizes, smells, skin colors, hair styles, bodily hair, makeup, perfumes, clothing styles, as well as objects they carry around with them (such as briefcases, books, jewelry, pens, combs, watches), and the objects people choose to decorate their environment with (clocks, paintings, furniture styles and colors, books, etc.). These artifactic messages have a strong influence on the initial perceptions and first impressions people have about others.

    Traditionally, health care practitioners have identified themselves through the use of easily recognizable artifactic cues, such as uniforms, equipment, and patient files. Health care uniforms are usually white (or light in color), symbolic of cleanliness and disinfection. Artifactic cues that providers use can have a profound effect on the judgments clients make about the providers competence and cleanliness. Attention to personal appearance, such as neatness and cleanliness of the uniform, grooming, and tasteful (moderate) use of jewelry, makeup, and perfumes can be important in convincing clients that a health care professional possesses all the knowledge and skills necessary to give effective treatment.

2. *Kinesics* include the way people move their bodies and position themselves, including postures, gestures, head nods, and leg movements. There are three basic types of gestures: *emblems*, which are gestures that have direct verbal translations such as nodding the head for yes and shaking the head for no, or waving the hand for hello; *illustrators*, which are gestures that accompany speech and accentuate what is being said, such as banging of hands on a table when the person speaking is angry; and *adaptors*, which are unconscious nervous gestures such as cracking the knuckles, scratching, or tapping the foot. Kinesic messages often indicate the level of someone's involvement in a given situation, as well as whether they are reacting positively or negatively to those around them.

Health care practitioners must be aware of their client's gestures simply for the fact that clients during treatment are often unable to express themselves through the use of words. Various emblem gestures are used to convey answers to questions by the practitioner such as, "Does this hurt? Are you comfortable?" Client adaptor gestures can often indicate their fear and tenseness (such as gripping the arms of the chair, or wringing their hands). Providers can use the information derived from these kinesic cues to direct responses to the client during treatment.

3. *Occulesics* consist of facial expressions and eye behaviors. The face is the primary emotional message-sending center of the human organism. Moreover, people monitor the facial expressions of others closely (as well as tracking their own facial expressions) to determine the emotions the face is expressing. Eye behavior includes eye-contact, gaze (direction, intensity, and duration), as well as blinking behaviors. Occulesic messages can tell us about the person's emotional state and level of interest in a situation or person.

The provider's face is a major source of emotional information for the client. Providers must constantly be aware of the expressions they present to the client, because clients are often watching while treatment is administered. If the provider's face communicates feelings of fear, surprise, anger, disgust, or contempt, it may cause the client to become unnecessarily nervous and fearful. As much as possible, try to smile and use other facial expressions to show support and interest. This will help alleviate client tension. Eye-contact is also an important part of occulesics in establishing rapport with the client. Maintaining eye-contact with clients and smiling pleasantly can communicate the provider's interest, respect, and caring for the person. Thoughtful and considerate use of occulesics can help clients feel more at ease in health care settings.

4. *Paralinguistics* are vocal cues accompanying speech, as well as environmental sounds. Vocal cues include the volume, pitch, tone, rate, and expression in someone's voice. Environmental sounds include music, wind, heavy machinery, train whistles, and so on. The vocal aspect of paralinguistics is the form of nonverbal communication that is most closely tied to verbal communication. Research has indicated that the tone of voice a health care professional uses with a client has a significant effect on the client's level of compliance (Milmoe, et al., 1967). The sounds surrounding us in our environment also affect the disposition and feelings of people.

Clients can often determine the provider's level of sincerity and caring for them more from the way the provider speaks to them than from what is actually said with words. Loud, rapid, forcefully spoken words can intimidate clients and communicate aggressiveness and even contempt. Soft, slow, expressionless speech may communicate disinterest in the client. It is usually best for providers to attempt to speak clearly (loudly enough for clients to hear all the words, but not loudly enough to frighten them) and expressively to hold patient interest and attention. Environmental sounds can either add to or detract from establishing a relaxed communication climate for clients.

5. *Tactilics* are touching behaviors, including self-touching, touching others, and the touching of objects. Skin-to-skin touching (*haptics*) is the most intimate form of touch. Research has indicated that human touch fulfills physiological and sociological needs for people (Montagu, 1971). An important need fulfilled by human touch that is related to health care practice is the expression of caring and empathy.

Health communication research has shown that touching behaviors in health care do not adequately meet client needs (Aguilera, 1967; Barnett, 1972; Day, 1973; Watson, 1975). Watson (1975) reported in a study of touch initiated by health care staff working in a geriatric facility that severely impaired clients were touched less often then those who were only mildly impaired, although those who were most ill were probably in great need of sensitive touch by health professionals (Watson, 1975). Moreover, this study showed that when practitioners did touch clients, they did so significantly more often for instrumental (job-related) purposes than for expressive (emotional) reasons (Watson, 1975). These research findings suggest that the health care practitioners' use of touch in this health care facility was not generally directed toward expressing empathy and caring for clients. It should be noted that this lack of touch can limit the effectiveness of health communication. In health care practice it is important to be able to touch clients in a sensitive and supportive way if they are in need of emotional support. Providers must, however, be careful to touch only clients who give cues that they are willing to accept being touched; a client should not feel as though his or her privacy has been invaded.

6. *Proxemics* is the study of the distance between people and objects, including the distances established in interpersonal relationships, group meetings, and environmental design. Each person maintains an expandable spatial bubble around himself or herself as an interpersonal buffer. This is referred to as *personal space*. We desire less personal space when we are comfortable with people in social situations and more personal space when we are uncomfortable. Personal space is a relational process. In a dyad, both communicators make personal space decisions and attempt to maintain "acceptable" boundaries of personal space. Sometimes your personal space expectations and the expectations of others conflict, and the result is spatial invasion. Spatial invasion makes people very uncomfortable and precipitates a communicative reaction of either fight or flight. Obviously, neither reaction is useful for the maintenance of healthy relationships. In health care practice, one must be careful to recognize and abide by the personal space expectations of others.

Another aspect of proxemics is territoriality. Territoriality differs from personal space in that it usually does not expand and contract in response to different situations and does not have to surround the person. People are territorial about their "possessions" or objects for which they claim ownership. These objects can range from smaller ones like clothing and books to major possessions such as homes and automobiles. People will generally protect their territory vigorously and will become quite angry if their territory is threatened or their possessions are taken from them. In medical organizations (like hospitals) where institutionalized clients are often denied many of their belongings such as clothing or jewelry, the clients may become upset and angry. The health practitioner should be careful in such cases to explain to clients why they cannot have these possessions and exactly how the institution is holding them in safekeeping. Possessions should not be removed unless absolutely necessary.

Still another part of the proxemic system of nonverbal communication is *small group ecology*, or the spatial arrangement of group members at meetings. Different spatial arrangements can have strong impact on the group communication that occurs at meetings. For example, it is easier to have a participative group discussion when members sit around a table or in a circle than it is if they sit in rows or are bunched haphazardly. Additionally, different group positions around a table tend to evoke different communication roles. For example, people who sit at the heads of the table are most likely to become group leaders, while people who flank the leaders (on either side) are likely to form coalitions with and support for the leaders. People sitting towards the middle of the table are likely to participate less in the group discussion. People will communicate more actively with one another if they are positioned face to face (*sociopetal orientation*), than if they are positioned away from one another (*sociofugal orientation*).

Architectural design and environmental planning also have a major impact on human communication. Open offices with glass windows through which people can see are more conducive for active communication than closed offices with walled in barriers to communication. Some modern health care organizations have designed facilities with movable walls and partitions (*semi-fixed space*) to elicit increased communication between members of health care teams who would have previously been separated from one another by unmovable walls and doors (*fixed space*). Moreover, the amount of space available to us in our immediate environment can affect our moods and attitudes. Small offices with low ceilings and no windows can cause people to feel boxed in and make them sullen and depressed, while cathedral ceilings and picture windows looking out on gardens and open spaces evoke feelings of peacefulness and contentment.

7. *Chronemics* deals with how time affects communication, including communication behaviors patterned over time, appointment keeping, and length of time communicating with others. Time is, perhaps, the form of nonverbal communication that people are least aware of, yet time has a major impact on human interaction. Human beings develop cyclical behavior patterns based on time of day, week, month, year, and so on. We depend on schedules and appointments to organize

our lives. The more time you spend communicating with others, regardless of the topic of conversation, the more you are telling them you believe they are important individuals. Conversely, the more time you keep people waiting to interact with you, the more you are implying they are insignificant to you. Health care practitioners often keep clients waiting without recognizing how the waiting time can work against the establishment of effective practitioner-client relationships. To counteract this perceptual problem, the health care professional should avoid keeping clients waiting. If a waiting period is inevitable, the practitioner should show respect for the client by explaining why the waiting period was necessary and expressing an apology.

Nonverbal communication is a very large and important part of the total human communication process. Each of the seven nonverbal systems includes a wide range of message types that affect innumerable communication situations. None of these nonverbal systems operates in isolation from other nonverbal systems, and nonverbal communication in general operates in concert with verbal communication. Knapp (1978) suggests, "Verbal and nonverbal communication should be treated as a total and inseparable unit" (p. 21). He describes six ways that nonverbal messages affect verbal messages in the total communication process, "Nonverbal behavior can repeat, contradict, substitute for, compliment, accent, or regulate verbal behavior." By developing sensitivity to the verbal and nonverbal messages human beings constantly encode and decode, the health care practitioner can learn both how to send the most appropriate messages to others and to interpret the variety of messages expressed consciously and unconsciously by clients and co-workers in health care situations.

Narrative Communication in Health Care

The *narrative paradigm* suggests that the telling of stories is a fundamental and universal human communication activity (Fisher, 1987; 1985; 1984; Lucaites & Condit, 1985). In fact, Fisher (1984) has referred to human beings as "homo narrans," tellers of stories. People tell stories to recount and account for their experiences, using narratives to organize and share with others their personal versions of social reality. Smith (1987) suggests, "It is through the telling of stories about ourselves and the events around us that we define reality, explain who we are to one another, and set the stage for future action" (p. 585). Stories also connect people to shared ideologies and logics by giving them a common means for interpreting and discussing history and life experiences, as well as by providing common frameworks for predicting the future.

Stories are a fundamental communication medium, a creative communication structure for connecting ideas together to make sense of what might otherwise be insensate (unconnected and confusing). Not only do stories make sense out of nonsense, but they can make sense in very entertaining, dramatic, exciting, educational, frightening, and/or humorous ways, thereby keeping an audience's attention and increasing the impact of the messages on the audience. We all can relate to a good story. That is why we have chosen to include so many case histories (stories) in this book. We believe that stories can bring concepts to life, can help to illustrate health care situations dramatically, and can enable readers to personally relate to the issues being presented in this book.

What attributes make a story a "good" story? Good stories are the ones that persist over time and are told and retold by and to different people. Good stories are entertaining and keep the listener's attention, causing the listener to think about the story and the implications of the story for his or her life. Fisher (1987) explains that good stories have narrative rationality and narrative probability, a sense of logic and the ring of truth. Smith (1987) explains that good stories are more complete than poor ones, provide more detail, are internally and externally consistent, and reveal the values of the story teller. Smith goes on to suggest that stories can be used to help address ethical issues in health care by enabling health care providers to learn about the values held by their clients that are imbedded in the stories these clients tell and by expressing their own values to consumers through the stories they tell or by elaborating on their clients' stories. (In chapter 8, Ethical Communication in Health Care, we will examine some of the contributions of narrative theory to illustrating ethical issues in health care).

In health care, stories are the ways in which people make sense of their personal health conditions. Stories are used by consumers of health care to explain to their doctors or nurses what their ailments are and how they feel about these health problems. Current health problems are connected symbolically to previous health conditions, as well as to beliefs about the health experiences of family members or friends, or to more general cultural beliefs about health. By listening to the stories a person tells about his or her health condition, the provider can learn a great deal about the person's cultural orientation, health belief system, and psychological orientation toward the condition.

Even though consumers' stories about personal health provide important health information for health care providers, health care providers often fail to evoke these personal narratives from consumers. Some health care providers are reticent about asking consumers to tell their stories, preferring not to get too "personal" with their clients. Some providers would rather just perform diagnostic tests and keep the interpersonal communication with their clients to a minimum. Some providers don't want to "waste" the time listening to stories. They would rather do most of the talking, even though listening is an essential diagnostic skill. By failing to encourage consumers to tell their stories, these providers are potentially losing a wealth of health information that would help them be more effective at providing health care to their clients.

Sometimes consumers may be hesitant about telling their health condition stories. They feel that their interpretations are not accurate or professional enough to share. These consumers should be encouraged to share their stories. They need to be told that their own interpretations of their health conditions are legitimate and important. By legitimizing consumers' personal narratives about their health, health care providers can validate the worth of individual consumers, encourage them to participate in their own health care, establish good working relationship with clients, and learn a great deal about physical and symbolic health conditions. After all, who is likely to know more about a person's health history and present condition than the actual person? Consumers can communicate insights into their emotional, psychological, and symbolic conditions by telling their stories to health care providers. Such information would be very difficult for providers to learn in any other way.

Health care providers can also use narratives to humanize health communication with clients and co-workers. Narratives about personal experiences, regardless of whether the stories concern health care issues or more general topics, can make health care providers appear to be more human and less distant to consumers. Clients have a tendency to stereotype and idealize health care providers based upon the professional roles providers perform; personal narratives help establish the relationship on a functional rather than a fictive basis. Stories are also good ways to emphasize important points health care providers want their clients to pay attention to and remember. Telling a newly diagnosed diabetic a story about how a former client misunderstood how to take his insulin and went into diabetic shock can really make an impression on the consumer and encourage him or her not to make the same mistake when administering his or her own insulin injections.

The stories we hear and tell about health care treatment are instrumental in the development of culturally-based health beliefs. Stories are important cultural dissemination media, socializing cultural members to interpret health and health care in similar culturally approved ways (Kreps, 1990d). The health beliefs we hold have powerful influences on health behaviors. By listening to the stories people tell about health and health care, we can learn about their cultural orientations to health. (We will discuss the importance of stories and culture in health care in Chapter 7).

Stories also perform many important communication functions in organizational life: reducing uncertainty, managing meanings, facilitating member bonding, and establishing (good and bad) reputations for organizations, organizational units, and organizational representatives (Brown, 1990; Kreps, 1990d). One of the best ways to learn about a complex organization is to listen to the stories that people tell about the organization (a hospital or a health care center, for example). You can learn a great deal about the formal and informal structure of the organization, the cultural values of the system, cultural heroes and villains within the system, and important underlying logics that are used within the organization for getting things done. In fact, Kreps (1990d) argues that analyzing the stories that are told about organizations is one of the best ways to gather relevant data about current organizational problems, constraints, and opportunities when directing organizational development efforts. (We will discuss the role of stories in organizational life more fully in chapter 5).

Summary

In this chapter we have explored the human communication process and have identified the major theories and principles of human communication that relate to the development of effective health communication skills. The most important propositions about the nature of human communication are listed below:

1. Human communication occurs when a person responds to a message and assigns meaning to it.
2. Human communication is a dynamic, ongoing process.
3. Human beings cannot not communicate.
4. In human communication, we simultaneously send and receive many messages on many different levels.
5. Human communication is bound to context and is irreversible.
6. Human communication is a transactional process.
7. Human communication is the primary tool people use to develop a sense of understanding about other people and situations.
8. All people are unique and their perceptions of reality and creations of meaning are unique.
9. Meanings are in people, not in words, objects or things.

10. Every message people send one another has both a content and a relationship dimension.
11. Personal communication shows respect for the person and tends to be a humanizing form of interaction.
12. Object communication shows disrespect and tends to be a dehumanizing form of interaction.
13. Feedback helps to clarify communication between people.
14. Rules of interaction are learned through metacommunication.
15. Verbal communication is a digital form of communication and is most effective at communicating content information.
16. Nonverbal communication is an analogic form of communication, and is most effective at communicating relationship information.
17. Language is an emergent phenomenon.
18. Verbal and nonverbal communication work together as a total, inseparable unit.
19. The telling of stories is a fundamental and universal human communication activity.
20. The stories people tell convey a great deal of information about their beliefs, values, and cultural orientations.

CHAPTER 3

The Interpersonal Health Communication Context

As a student, I had an experience with a patient, Mr. Burns, that I've never forgotten. When Mr. Burns found out he had high blood pressure, he simply wouldn't believe it. "Change my diet? Never!" he vowed and turned his back on the nursing team gathered around his bed. I was shocked, yet fascinated, by his behavior. How could an intelligent man like Mr. Burns defy sound medical advise?

Every day I spent a few extra minutes getting to know him better. We chatted about the ball team. We talked about his family. We even touched on the effect of his illness insofar as he might have to reduce his work hours. But neither of us so much as whispered the word diet.

By the week's end, we were greeting one another like old friends.

And when I least expected it, Mr. Burns turned to me like a woebegone child and asked, "Am I really going to have to quit eating fried chicken?"

"You might." I answered softly, patting his arm.

"But I don't want to," he wailed.

In simple terms, I told Mr. Burns about the effect of fried foods on people with high blood pressure. This time, he listened intently.

When I finished speaking, Mr. Burns, with a shake of his head, said, "Stewed chicken will never replace Kentucky Fried. But I guess I could give it a try."

Later, while I was telling my supervisor about our conversation, I realized with pleasure that I'd been practicing the good communication techniques I'd been taught in class. I cared about Mr. Burns. I wanted to help him feel better about himself and, if possible, help him to establish a trusting relationship. I'd been able to get through to Mr. Burns. Me — a lowly student.

Communicating isn't so difficult, I realized. But it must be more than reciting verbal techniques. When a health care practitioner really cares about her patient, she should try to ensure an honest exchange of feelings.

The lesson had such an impact on me that I've built my career around the importance of practicing good communications (adapted from Mercer, no date.).

The Health Communication System

This chapter will focus on effective one-to-one relationships in health care. However, before we isolate such interpersonal communication, we want to remind you that no communication takes place in a vacuum. Human beings are always involved with each other in the communication process and *all communication takes place within a system.* The individual can be seen at the center of the system (See Figure 3.1). The individual client is surrounded by health care providers in the next ring, forming the practitioner-client relationship. The client and the health care providers interact within the hospital or other health care setting (third ring); the particular health care setting functions within the community (fourth ring); the community is part of the environment which includes state and national organizations. It is not possible to construct a model which would include all parts of the system ad infinitum, but this analogy indicates the importance of understanding the impact and interrelatedness of all the various components on the individual.

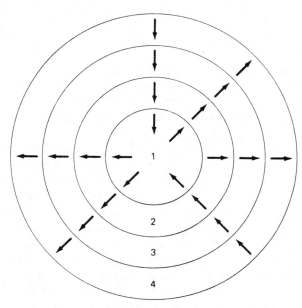

1. The Individual
2. Health Care Practitioners
3. Health Care Setting
4. Outside Environment

Figure 3.1   The Client's Health Communication System

Closed systems are ones in which little or no information, interaction, or exchange takes place within or between parts of the system. A closed system can be compared to an autocratic family in which there is one head of the household; family members' activities are structured around the family unit, and little information comes to the family from outside. A totally closed system could not continue to exist because outside forces will eventually intrude either because some family members will rebel and welcome outside input or because the person in control will need information or services not available in the family unit. Certain systems will find various degrees of openness or closedness advantageous. A closed health care system, for example, has a clear line of command. There is little question of control or of what duties are assigned to various professionals. New and threatening information which challenges the system is not allowed. An *open system*, on the other hand, has no rigid structure and is open to information from other systems and subsystems. Thus, it is constantly changing. While that change can often be beneficial, it is threatening to the status quo and can cause upheaval. In order for a health system to stay "healthy," it must utilize advantages from both the open and closed approaches.

The context of an interaction that occurs among members of the system, particularly the practitioner-client relationship, is complex because of the interrelatedness described above. A fictional client named McGrady is at the center of a system that incorporates many relationships. Her relationship with Nurse Bruins is an *interpersonal or dyadic one.* Client McGrady also has relationships with other members of the health care team whom she sees sometimes as a group and sometimes individually. Further, she has relationships with other organizations in the environment. For example, she deals with her Medicaid representative and her state legislator in order to get better health care. Her relationships constantly change due to the number of people participating to varying degrees in every interaction.

Whether McGrady is in an open or closed system will affect her care and how she receives information about that care. In a closed system, she will clearly understand the hierarchy of her care, although there will be limited information exchange. In an open system, much more interaction will take place. The relatedness of interpersonal relationships in systems is provided not only to emphasize the complexity of communication but to provide a background for understanding the unique and complicated practitioner-client relationship and to underscore the fact that it functions within a much larger system.

Practitioner-Client Relationships

The practitioner-client relationship has been a major topic in recent health care literature. Writers discuss such factors as the unequal power relationship between practitioners and clients (Mendelsohn, 1981), as well as the mythology of health settings which makes communication more confusing and complex (Barnlund, 1976; Booth, 1983). Double messages are often given to clients in health care. For example, the dentist giving a shot to a child might say, "This doesn't hurt." In fact, it does hurt. The dentist's statement contradicts the child's physical sensations, and the child is put in a situation of deciding which to believe. The dentist's message is thus antithetical to good communication. Knowing how to deal with discomfort without creating double messages is a crucial skill for health care professionals (Dangott, Thornton and Page, 1978).

Double messages put people into *double-bind* situations; they receive contradictory communication which confuses the situation. Jargon creates a double-bind for the practitioner. While jargon may help the physician provide accurate instructions and diagnoses to other health colleagues, it confuses and sometimes frightens the client. Jargon, which was discussed in detail in chapter 2, also contributes to a closed interpersonal communication system where information is not exchanged.

Double-binds also result from labelling health care clients. For example, many times the label "difficult" is applied to the person who is educated about an illness, who knows enough to ask intelligent questions, and who will occasionally refuse to undergo certain treatments or tests. This scenario is often compounded when treatment is not working and the health care practitioner blames the lack of success on the client's "difficultness" (Bandler and Grinder, 1975).

In contrast, health care practitioners who work toward congruent and productive relationships report that with good communication, problems can be more readily diagnosed, clients can be more easily satisfied, and the work setting can be enhanced for the health professional. The case used at the beginning of the chapter illustrates how communication can enhance a health care relationship and help to facilitate the cooperation so vitally needed between health care providers and consumers.

Establishing an Effective Contract

Strong interpersonal relationships are based upon the fulfillment of needs by relational partners. Each partner in a dyadic relationship expects the other to act in specified ways. The key to establishing effective relationships is to make expectations clear.

In marital relationships, for example, there are many mutual expectations about the appropriate interpersonal behaviors of the husband and the wife. The husband might expect the wife to wash the dishes, and the wife might expect the husband to vacuum the carpet. Often, however, these expectations remain unspoken. Each relational partner might think that the other should know what is expected without being told. When marriage partners are unaware or unsure of each other's expectations, there is a high probability they will not act in accord with each other's wishes. To complicate this situation further, the expectations relational partners have for one another change constantly, making the potential for the fulfillment of these expectations even less likely. The same expectations that hold for marital contracts hold for the "contract" between the client and the health care practitioner.

Inevitably, when people fail to meet the expectations of others, they disappoint those persons and weaken those relationships. Behaviors that fail to meet relational expectations are interpreted negatively. It is often assumed that the person who is not fulfilling the expectations is doing so because he or she is either mad or bad. Mad or bad interpretations imply that the noncompliant individual is mad (crazy or stupid) or bad (purposefully uncooperative). Mad or bad interpretations foster suspicion and mistrust within the relationship. The more communicators fail to meet the expectations of those with whom they are in a relationship, the more the relationship is weakened. Communicators are frustrated by the negative responses they receive and are often unaware they are violating others' expectations. The failure to meet others' expectations can instigate inappropriate, often angry and retaliatory, responses. These behaviors, in turn, instigate additional inappropriate behaviors, all of which fail to meet relational expectations, causing a vicious cycle of escalating relational deterioration. For example, a client kept waiting for hours might refuse to pay a bill for months or decide to stop seeing the professional without explanation.

To a certain extent effective relationships are very much like contractual agreements. They aren't exactly explicit legal contracts such as the contract used in business arrangements. Relationships are usually less formal than legal contracts, generally taking the form of unspoken implicit contracts. Such a contract implies that communicators should act in certain ways toward one another. For example in a friendship relationship between two nurses working together in the emergency room of a hospital, the implicit contract established might call for informal and playful interaction between the two individuals. The two nurses might tease one another or use lighthearted bantering as a means of relieving some of the tension and stress of their work in the emergency room. This is an implicit contract because it is not formally required by the organization or formally agreed upon by the nurses. The relationship evolves informally out of past interactions between the nurses. The nurses unspoken agreement to continue fulfilling each other's expectations for light-hearted interaction is an implicit contract.

Effective interpersonal relationships both in and out of health care settings have clearly understood implicit contracts between relational partners. Not only are the communicators aware of the expectations they have of one another, but they work at continually updating their perceptions of each other's expectations. These communicators try to update their awareness of the implicit contract by giving and seeking interpersonal feedback which enables them to continue to act appropriately with one another as their relationship grows.

Therapeutic Relationships

Interpersonal relationships have many different functions. They can provide communicators with excitement, support, friendship, love, financial gain, and intellectual stimulation — as well as serving to increase or decrease their overall state of health. The more therapeutic interpersonal communication is, the more the communication helps individuals involved increase their levels of health.

Therapeutic communication has been defined in many different ways. Fuller and Quesada (1973) expressed the clinical perspective on therapy when they described therapeutic communication as "the characteristics of information exchange between therapist and patient that facilitate a mutually gratifying relationship between participants so as to accomplish the primary goal of reduced morbidity for the patient." Their approach to therapeutic communication suggests that it is accomplished only by formally designated "therapists" to help "patients" to prolong their lives. This is a fairly restrictive perspective on therapeutic communication that fails to recognize the wider application of therapy in everyday life.

Pettegrew (1977) has broadened the Fuller and Quesada approach to therapeutic communication by identifying a larger range of therapeutic outcomes, although he maintains a somewhat clinical perspective when he defines therapeutic communication as, "the verbal and paraverbal communication transactions between a helper and a helpee which results in feelings of psychological (thoughts), emotional (feelings), and or physical (actions) relief by the helpee" (p. 595). Barnlund further liberates the perspective of therapeutic communication, expanding the range of settings, participants, and applications of therapeutic communication when he explains that interpersonal relationships "are regarded as therapeutic when they provide personal insight or reorientation, and when they enable persons to participate in more satisfying ways in future social encounters" (Barnlund, 1968).

Barnlund's approach to therapeutic communication does not limit its application to trained health practitioners, nor does it limit it to health care practice and the preservation of human life. His approach implies that any individual has the potential for communicating therapeutically by helping another person to understand himself or herself more fully, thereby aiding that individual in deciding how to direct behaviors to best achieve needs and goals. Furthermore, according to this perspective on therapeutic communication, interpersonal feedback is therapeutic if it informs people about others' perceptions of them, offering a clearer image about the reactions people have to their communication. Ultimately, therapeutic communication enable individuals to communicate more effectively to achieve their personal goals.

A key health care function of interpersonal relationships is the provision of mutual social support between relational partners (Albrecht and Adelman, 1987; Cohen and Syme, 1985; Frosland, Brodsky, Olson & Stewart, 1979; Gottlieb, 1981). Interpersonal communication between relational partners has great potential for therapeutic benefits through providing relevant and supportive content and relationship information. The provision of therapeutic communication is not just limited to trained health care professionals nor is it offered only during health care practice; anyone has the potential to communicate therapeutically (Kreps, 1981). For example, hairdressers and bartenders often provide their clients with therapeutic counsel (Cowen, et al., 1979; Cowen, McKim and Weissberg, 1981; Wiesefeld and Weiss, 1979). All interpersonal relationships are potentially therapeutic to the extent that interactants provide one another with informative feedback leading to enlightenment and redirection (Burke, Weir, and Duncan, 1976).

Certainly all interpersonal communication is not therapeutic. Interpersonal communication can often have nontherapeutic effects by confusing and frustrating communicators rather than helping them achieve personal insight and reorientation. Popular evidence about the growing frustrations and dissatisfactions experienced by people involved in the health care system (discussed in chapter 1) seems to indicate that much interpersonal communication in health care is nontherapeutic. Nontherapeutic communication is counterproductive to the goals of health care because it fosters dissatisfaction among communicators and undermines the spirit of cooperation that is essential to effective health care relationships.

Watzlawick, Beavin and Jackson (1967) have identified several situations where interpersonal relationships can become "pathological" due to nontherapeutic communication. Pathologies are defined as ". . . disturbances that can develop in human communication," and therapeutic communication functions to ameliorate pathologies. Similarly, Ruesch (1957) has differentiated between therapeutic communication and disturbed communication, suggesting that human communication can range on a continuum from highly therapeutic to highly disturbed (nontherapeutic). Therapeutic communication can be used in many different health care situations to help individuals grow and adapt, increasing their sense of satisfaction with themselves and with their interpersonal relationships.

Rossiter and Pearce (1975) have described honesty and validation as two key characteristics of therapeutic communication; they contend "that honesty accompanied by validation results in psychological growth for persons and that the lack of honesty and validations is likely to retard psychological growth and possibly bring about psychological deterioration." Truax and Carkhuff (1967) have identified three key characteristics demonstrated by therapeutic communicators that are similar to those offered by Rossiter and Pearce. Their characteristics include: 1) accurate empathy and understanding; 2) nonpossessive warmth and respect; 3) genuineness and authenticity. Rogers (1957) has described therapeutic communication characteristics similarly, identifying such attributes as genuineness and congruence, unconditional positive regard, and empathic understanding. A combination and synthesis of the characteristics of therapeutic communicators advocated by these theorists (Rossiter and Pearce, 1975; Truax and Carkhuff, 1967; and Rogers, 1957) indicates the importance of the following communicator characteristics in communicating therapeutically: *empathy, trust, honesty, validation (confirmation) and caring.*

Empathy refers to the ability to develop a full understanding of another person's condition and feelings and to relate that understanding to the person. Health communicators can demonstrate empathy for another person by accurately stating and acknowledging the other's feelings in interpersonal interaction. Often, empathy can be shown nonverbally as well as verbally. Nodding one's head when the other person reveals something about him or herself confirms that the information has been understood. Maintaining eye contact with the individual speaking and mirroring the person's facial expressions in a genuine manner is another sign of confirmation. In health care interviews, mirror questions and reflective probes (discussed later in this chapter) can help communicate empathy by letting the interviewee know the practitioner is following and understanding what is being said.

Empathy is an important part of the patient-provider relationship and can even affect the accuracy of information sharing. Training programs to identify and teach empathy to nurses, physicians and other health care providers have been developed. Empathy is also a useful tool in assisting patients to work through their problems. There is some evidence that nonverbal communication is linked to empathy and health care (Hardin & Halares, 1983).

Trust is a belief that a person will respect another's needs and desires and will behave towards him or her in a responsible and predictable manner. Trusting behaviors are those that ". . . deliberately increase a person's vulnerability to another person" (Rossiter & Pearce, 1975). In establishing a trusting relationship, it may be necessary for one person to take a chance by disclosing information about himself or herself to another that might make him or her more vulnerable to that person. If the other person responds responsibly, and perhaps discloses some risky information of his or her own, the chances that trust will develop are good. If, however, an individual reacts irresponsibly or inappropriately to another's self disclosure trust will not develop. Due to the risk involved in establishing trusting relationships, trust is most often established little by little over long periods of time. In health care, due to the intensity of many interpersonal situations, trust can sometimes be established or destroyed rather quickly depending on the appropriateness of the communicative response.

Trust in health care is an important variable for communicating about uncomfortable topics and is also important between health care providers

(Northouse, 1979). It is the foundation of human relationships and successful health care intervention (Caserta 1989).

Honesty refers to the ability to communicate truthfully, frankly, and sincerely. There is never total honesty in any situation, because there is never total truth. People perceive the world according to their own view of reality; often people perceive the world very differently from one another. Honest communication, however, does not imply objective truth but subjective truth. It is not purposely deceptive but is intended to be a truthful representation of information as the individual knows it. "A person communicates honestly to the extent that his messages accurately express his awareness of his experience and invite the listener to share in that experience" (Rossiter & Pearce, 1975). Honest self-disclosure in health care relationships implicitly invites reciprocal honesty by relational partners. Honesty or truth telling is also discussed in chapter 8.

Validation or confirmation occurs when a communicator feels as though other communicators accept and respect what he or she has to say. Validating communication affirms the worth of the person and his or her experiences. (Validation and confirmation is similar to personal communication discussed in depth in chapter 2). To validate other people doesn't mean agreeing totally with everything they say but respecting their right to express their opinions and taking what they have to say seriously. Validating or confirming communication tends to humanize interaction. It tells the person with whom you are talking that you are willing to be influenced by what they say and that their communication is important to you. Health communicators can validate and confirm one another in interpersonal communication by listening carefully to what is being said and responding to the other's messages congruently.

Validating communication is often referred to as confirming behavior. *Confirming communicators* use some of the following behaviors; they give direct responses; nod; show verbal and nonverbal interest; express agreement, disagreement and neutrality; expand, explore and express feelings; or request clarification.

Nonconfirming behaviors include the use of irrelevant comments, giving ambiguous responses and interruptions. Failing to acknowledge others, the use of impersonal language, shifting the focus of conversation to something tangential, restless nonverbal clues and demeaning and disparaging remarks are also disconfirming (Heineken, 1983).

Paul Watzlawick and others (1967) stressed that confirming behavior is necessary for healthy mental development and emotional stability. Disconfirming behavior, which conveys the feeling to the listener that he or she does not exist, is psychologically damaging.

Confirming behavior is particularly important in health care (Watzlawick,

Beavin & Jackson, 1967 and Heineken & Roberts, 1983). Heineken (1983) linked disconfirming behaviors with unhealthy mental states of patients as well as lower self-esteem and dysfunctional patterns of communication.

The research on confirmation and validation suggests that health care providers practice confirming behaviors under supervision and become aware of the importance that confirming behavior holds for patients and for other health care providers (Heineken, 1980; Heineken & Roberts, 1983).

Caring refers to the level of emotional involvement communicators express for one another. It is what Rogers calls "unconditional positive regard," the demonstration of interest and concern for the other person's well-being. Caring communication must be sincere and appropriate to be useful in health care. Communicators can express caring for one another nonverbally by paying attention to what the other person is saying (maintaining eye contact and nodding when appropriate), exhibiting emotionally congruent facial expressions, and by using their vocal and tactile behaviors to show supportiveness. Health communicators can demonstrate caring for one another by expressing genuine concern over the other's problems and communicating a willingness to help the other person work through his or her hardships.

Caring has become a key word in health care. In his controversial book *What Kind of Life*, which attempts to set limits on health care, Dan Callahan (1990) argues that primacy in health care needs to be given to caring over curing. The importance of the lay view of what caring means is stressed by Kitsen (1987). Unfortunately, health care practitioners often have difficulty in differentiating between instructing and caring (Lane, 1983). Recently, caring has been associated with women's styles of relationships, although advocates of caring behavior argue that it should be adapted by both sexes (Gilligan, 1982; Kreps, 1990; Nodding, 1984).

Each of the five characteristics of therapeutic communication (empathy, trust, honesty, validation, and caring) are important skills for effective health communication. In many situations the five overlap and merge with one another. For example, empathy and caring can be expressed with the same nonverbal messages of eye contact and head nods; validation, honesty, and caring are also reciprocally occurring human communication behaviors. That is, the expression of empathic, trusting, honest, validating, or caring communications generally induces a reciprocal expression by others. Due to this reciprocity, the use of therapeutic communication in health care can encourage others to communicate similarly, resulting in a spiraling or building effect in therapeutic communication.

In addition to the five characteristics of therapeutic communication, the authors of this book would like to emphasize the importance of humor and listening in health care interaction. The use of humor to reduce stress in health professionals underpinned television series such as "M.A.S.H." and "St. Elsewhere." Humor in high stress situations is often cathartic among health care professionals; it relieves the strain. A new hospital in one of our communities is gambling that even the emergency room needs humor because they put floor to ceiling murals of scenes from "M.A.S.H." all over the emergency waiting room walls. Norman Cousins also argued that humor is useful toward neutralizing stress and changing the meaning of situations so they are less stressful. While cruel or inappropriate jokes are certainly out of place in the therapeutic interaction, gentle humor can be useful in any human exchange (Cousins, 1979).

Listening is an integral part of therapeutic communication and it is reflected in the caring process. Harlem (1977) emphasizes the importance and difficulty of listening to clients. He says:

> When I was in practice, I found the most exhausting and exacting part of communication was listening to patients, not only to the apparent verbal meaning of what they wanted me to know, or believe and why. It involved trying to enter the patient's world each time, empathizing with him, and reading his body language, those unconscious and often telltale, gestures, mannerisms and expressions (p. 5).

We have adapted the ten classic mistakes made in listening from the work of Ralph Nichols (1957) a national expert on listening skills. Every health practitioner should read these questions carefully and consciously decide whether they, as individuals, are guilty of one or more of these listening errors:

1. Do you tend to avoid discussing difficult material with clients, particularly material which takes time and thought?

2. Do you pretend to listen or show interest when your mind is elsewhere?

3. Do you dismiss the clients discussion as uninteresting? Hearing about headaches at least 20 times a day is taxing on the health provider. However, headache symptoms can mask other problems. Effective listening requires attention, patience and resisting the urge to control the conversation.

4. Are you easily distracted? Distractions are always present in health related settings. Whenever possible, space and time should be designed to eliminate distractions when one-to-one interaction is necessary to develop a good relationship with a client.

5. Do you find fault with the way the patients, talk, dress or act? Focusing on ancillary factors can divert your attention from what is being said.

6. Do you listen only for facts or details? If so, you might be failing to take the emotions, behaviors and intentions of the client into consideration which would give you the real clues as to what is happening.

7. Do you become angry at what the speaker is saying, particularly if they are upset about health care or the way you run your office?

8. If the client uses emotional language does that antagonize you? If so, you might become defensive and not hear what is being said.

9. Do you become preoccupied with your note taking? Note-taking is recognized as important for both the health care practitioner and the client, but it can also be an avoidance technique. Listen and make eye contact before you write.

10. Do you become distracted because it is taking the client a long time to speak? Most people speak at approximately 125 words a minute but are capable of listening to 500 spoken words. In order to really hear what is being said, it is important to learn to concentrate, since it is easy to become distracted.

Good listeners give reflective feedback, indicating to the speaker whether his or her message is being understood. This is accomplished by asking questions, making statements and by offering visual cues that indicate whether or not you have understood what is being said. Eighty to ninety-two percent of all communication is estimated to be nonverbal, and your eye contact and use of body language will be clues to the speaker that you understand what he or she is saying. Your posture, the way you lean and where you sit or stand indicates interest or lack of interest in what your colleague or client is saying. It is important not to rehearse what you plan to say. Instead concentrate on what is being said.

Listening is of paramount importance in the operating room (Keelan & Stokoe, 1983), home health care and during the health care interview (Stewart & Roter, 1989; Talento & Crockett-McKeever, 1983).

The Health Care Interview

The initial dialogue between the practitioner and the client usually takes the form of an interview. Interviews can be seen as formal consultations or mutual viewings of data. In the health care setting, interviews are usually a formal and encompassing means of consultation between practitioners and clients. The perception of the interview by the various participants has a great deal to do with its success. Whereas the traditional interview has long been thought of as the "doctor-client interview," there is now an awareness in health care that all members of the health care team participate in the interview process at some time during client care. The following discussion should be helpful to all health care personnel, as well as to consumers of health care who would like to improve the consultations they have with health care practitioners. The suggestions given for effective interviewing should be incorporated with the elements of therapeutic communication in order to be most useful.

In planning the interview, the topic of the next section, listening to the client's stories, particularly through a nondirective approach, should be given serious consideration. A case study which gives some direction in how to use this approach is presented by Sharf (1990). Another particularly useful edited book that pertains to the medical interview is *Communication with Medical Patients*, by Stewart & Roter (1989).

Preparing for the Interview

The first part of the interview process is to establish the goal of the interview for both the interviewer (usually the health care practitioner) and the interviewee (usually the client). Generally, the interview takes place because the client is seeking help and the practitioner needs information in order to provide that help. Traditionally, health care practitioners have used a directive approach as their primary interview style. The *directive interview* is a tightly controlled process used to obtain specific information and to provide the proper course of action that the interviewee should take. The implication of the directive interview is that the client is incapable of identifying the problem or of aiding in the selection of the best solution. There are many problems with the traditional directive interview. Often the client might not agree with the prescribed regimen or might feel isolated from the suggested solution to the medical problem. Clients have also reported that the practitioner did not hear all of what he or she was trying to express (Enelow & Swisher, 1972).

In the *client-centered interview* based on the theories of Carl Rogers (1951), the practitioner's role is that of a helper who tries to assist the client in achieving his or her own insights and solutions to problems. The client-centered interview is sometimes referred to as a nondirective approach and is the antithesis of the traditional directive approach. In the client-centered interview, the interviewer reflects back to the interviewee information he or she has provided — giving the interviewee the opportunity to correct any misperceptions. The notion behind this approach is each person is his or her best expert. Offering encouragement to explore ideas and feelings about self will help individuals solve their own problems. In health care, this may become difficult for clients because they often do not know how to express or describe health care symptoms. They may not always have the expertise to diagnose or solve complex health care problems. The solution to this problem is, of course, to take the best of the directive interview and the client-centered interview methods in order to build a model to fit the client's needs.

One way to use a client-centered approach is to listen to a client's story as it is told. The behavioral sciences have recently had an increased interest in narrative theory (discussed in chapter 2). Narrative theory or the chronicle given by a participant in his or her own words with little or no prodding is particularly important for the health care interview. In any interview, there are two stories or points of view: the story of the interviewer and the interviewee. These stories arise out of different belief systems where the health practitioner's beliefs involve the world of medicine and the patient's beliefs involve the values about illness that he or she has learned from culture.

The interview process should not only take these two different perspectives or belief systems into consideration but should be aware that "the story of an illness — the patient's history — has two protagonists: the body and the person" (Cassell, 1985). The tasks of the interviewer are to define the nature of the problem, to establish the goals of treatment and to identify the roles which will be assumed by the doctor and the client.

In addition to determining and identifying the kind of interview (directive or nondirective) that will take place, practitioners and clients should identify goals such as the timing of the interview and the kinds of questions that will be asked and answered in order to establish the nature of the problem. Additionally, interviewers will want to be aware of interview style as well as techniques. Probably the most important goal of the interviewer is to remember that involving the client in his or her own care from the outset of the initial interview will insure a more effective treatment. Health care practitioners are particularly encouraged to incorporate videotaping in their interview techniques (Taleno & Crocket-McKeever, 1983).

Time

As we discussed in the nonverbal communication section of chapter 2, chronemics is an important nonverbal aspect of communication. Time will probably affect the interview more than any other factor. The health practitioner as well as the client will make initial judgements of each other based partially on respective treatments of the time dimension. The use or misuse of time can become an obstacle if either party is kept waiting for too long; they will lose trust or respect for the other (Benjamin, 1981). Cline (1990) reports the findings of Frankel and Beckmann that only 23 percent of patients are able to tell their doctor all their complaints and that physicians listen for only 18 seconds before interrupting (Dreyfuss, 1986).

Pluchman (1978) also discussed the issue of time in the health setting. She notes that a time contract between practitioner and client is often one-sided on behalf of the provider. At the time of the scheduling of the interview and again when the interview begins, a realistic contract regarding time should be established to provide a framework for the interview. If time constraints and/or emergency interruptions indicate that the interview is going to be a short one, parties to the medical interview have a right to know so that they can structure their questions and answers accordingly. If the duration of the interview is known, less repetition is less likely. If time is frankly discussed, both the beginning and the ending of the interview will be structured more efficiently. If other interviews regarding health problems are going to take place in the future, this should also be made clear. The thoughtful, organized health care practitioner will schedule initial interviews at an appropriate time of day when emergencies are less likely to occur. Interviews conducted when there are too many distractions or when the participants are tired will not be successful and the appropriate information will not be obtained. Proper planning and use of time can conserve usable energy.

Practitioners argue that there simply aren't enough hours in the day or that emergencies often interfere with the ideal time constraints of a client's appointment. Clients, on the other hand, often feel that there is not enough time to discuss problems in detail with the practitioner or that the practitioner is too intent on making money or fulfilling quotas to take the necessary time to listen to concerns. Additionally, members of either group might be *monochronic*. That is, they are clockwatching people intent on being on time, while *polychronic* people are more relationship-oriented and conclude a prior interaction (despite possibly being late) before they begin a new one (Pluchman, 1978).

The quality of communication directly affects the degree of medical success. Although communication is time consuming, a satisfactory client-practitioner relationship can prevent law suits (Gorney, 1988) and dissatisfaction (Cline, 1990).

Space

Space is also an important variable in the interview situation. We are constantly arranging ourselves in relation to others in some spatial context.

Space as an internal, nonverbal message source can seriously affect communication. Where we sit, how much we distance ourselves from clients, and the arrangement of the office or other health care setting are of great importance. Spatial distances, as studied by anthropologist Edward T. Hall, give us some idea of how much area people in our Western culture need to operate efficiently. Space is often related to culture as we indicate in chapter 7, and because health practitioners see a vast array of people from many cultures, it is important that they be aware of the client's spatial needs. This can be done by observing the client to see if distances are comfortable or not. Additionally, the interviewer can ask the client where he or she would like to sit or place his or her belongings. In interviews in which the practitioner wants self-disclosure to take place, it is often more acceptable to sit beside the desk rather than behind it so that space and objects do not become barriers.

A disturbance related to space is illustrated by Pluchman (1978). The verbal statement, "I'm not afraid of contracting your disease," accompanied by the health practitioner standing a substantial distance from the client would be perceived as a confusing and incongruent message. Kelly (1972) found that practitioners were believed, liked, and trusted when they sat close.

Space should also be considered in terms of territorial behavior. Clients, like most people, often exhibit territorial behavior regarding their clothes and their bodies. During physical exams where clients are asked to disrobe, the perceptive interviewer should be aware of privacy needs and should set up the interview situation so there will be no interruptions (Pluchman, 1978).

Developing the Interaction

After time and space guidelines are established, other parameters of the interview should also be discussed. Clients should be given a short overview regarding what will happen. This should include the kinds of questions that will be asked as well as the kinds of procedures that might be used if the interview is combined with an examination. The practitioner needs to obtain some idea of the language constraints of the client. Is the client aware of medical terms such as penis or vagina if those terms are relevant to the interview? Does the use of those terms embarrass the client? While these kinds of questions should, of course, not be asked at the beginning of the interview, the interviewer should keep the level of information exchange in mind and be aware of the client's comfort level (Braverman, 1990). Clients should never be patronized. They should be addressed in language they clearly understand. The health care practitioner should also be aware of both verbal and nonverbal cues (Geist & Hardesty, 1990). Ballard-Reish (1990) present a model of participative decision making in which good communicators can review their rights and responsibilites so that communication can take place effectively.

As the practitioner-client relationship develops, and possibly in the first interview, truth telling can become an issue. For example, if the client states that he thinks he has lung cancer and wants to know the probabilities of survival from that disease, a decision regarding truth telling must be made. (While not the principal element in the initial interview, it will become increasingly important as the health care relationship continues.) Much of the literature of informed consent and truth-telling advocates honest and open discussion for most health care problems but the individual health care provider must determine his or her own stance. Additionally, it is most important to determine the client's point of view. This can best be done by an open discussion of the issue during one of the interviews. Practitioners sometimes make the assumption that clients do or do not want to know the truth with little data from the client. Chapter 8 will discuss truth telling and ethics in health care in more detail.

Winning the client's confidence is important in the interview process. This can be done by showing interest, respecting attitudes and ideas, and by stressing the client's physical or mental strengths. It is important not to pry but to let the client choose the rate and amount of self-disclosure.

Interviewers should not probe deeply into subjects for which they are not qualified. For example, if the client wants to discuss a serious sexual problem and the health provider has little or no training in this area, the client should not be encouraged to share potentially embarrassing and private data that is not pertinent to the professional's area of expertise and which will have to be repeated to the next professional. It is appropriate in this situation for the practitioner to tell the client that sexuality (or other relevant topic) is not the provider's area but that he or she will be happy to put the client in touch with the appropriate person.

Watching and listening for nonverbal communication clues is crucial. For example, excessive perspiration or wringing of the hands can be viewed as signs of nervousness, at which point the interview can be redirected until the interviewee is more comfortable. Interviewers are often nervous about the interview, failing to utilize the chronemic (time) aspects of interviewing effectively. Health care practitioners generally overestimate the length of silent pauses by their clients. Just as silent pauses in conversation cause many people discomfort on a first date, they can cause providers and clients to become uncomfortable. Pauses in interpersonal conversation are natural and shouldn't be avoided. In fact, in health care interviews, clients often may need to pause to in order to interpret their ideas, feelings, and symptoms before communicating this information to the health care provider.

The health care interview is an important interpersonal communication setting for the exchange of content and relationship information between providers and consumers (Benjamin, 1981; Cline, 1983; Roter & Hall, 1986). An important communication function of the interview is to initiate the development of effective health care relationships and the development of provider and consumer health communication rules. The relational messages which interview participants send one another establish the guidelines for an implicit contract between the health care provider and the health care consumer. In effective interviews, care is taken by practitioners to put clients at ease so they feel comfortable about sharing personal health information and are receptive to health information provided to them. Interview participants also depend upon their interpersonal messages to elicit full and clear content information, to explore treatment options, and to make informed health care decisions (Ballard-Reisch, 1990).

Traditionally, health care providers are charged with the responsibility of maintaining control of the interview by keeping it focused, establishing rapport with the client by communicating in a sensitive and caring manner, and bringing closure to the interview by responding to client questions and clearly explaining future health care activities (Foley & Sharf, 1981).

Health care consumers, despite their personal stake in the health care situation, are not routinely given, nor do they often take, opportunities to control health care interviews by directing questions to their providers and voicing their concerns and suggestions about health care treatments (Greenfield, Kaplan & Ware, 1985). If interview participants can coordinate the exchange of content and relationship information and make the information exchange more effective, the health care interview can provide them with a structured setting for gathering relevant health information and establishing effective provider/consumer relationships (Carroll & Monroe, 1980; Cassata, 1983).

Interview Questions

It is important not to have a cookbook formula for the interview. Each client and each professional needs an individual approach. However, the interviewer should be familiar with different approaches and types of questions. An *open-ended question* is one which allows the client to answer without much direction. For example, the questions "How do you feel?" or "What is the matter with you today?" do not direct the answer. Instead they invite the client to give his or her perceptions, views, opinions, thoughts, and feelings. Often an open-ended question can lead to good rapport (Benjamin, 1981). Open questions do have some disadvantages. For example, answers might give superfluous information or take more time than is allocated. *Closed questions* limit options and sometimes specify answers to the questions themselves. They are restrictive by nature. For example, a *moderately closed question* might be, "How long has it been since your last physical?" An example of a *highly closed question* would be to ask the client to pick one of four given answers.

Bi-polar questions are a common type of closed question often used and misused in the interview process. In this type of question, the respondent is limited to one of two choices: "Do you drink or not?" "Do you approve or disapprove of birth control?" The assumptions undergirding bi-polar questions are that there are only two possible answers and that they are totally in opposition to each other (Stewart & Cash, 1978).

The advantage of closed questions is that the interviewer can control the questions and answers more effectively and that he or she can ask more questions in more areas in less time. It is easier to record and tally answers on closed questions. Disadvantages of the closed questions are that the wrong kind of information can be given and that too little data is obtained. The answers to closed questions often fail to reveal feelings or attitudes which might be pertinent to the client's health problem. Additionally, closed questions might force certain positions too early in the interview. These disadvantages and others make the use of the closed question a delicate tool in the hands of the practitioner.

Other kinds of questions which can be asked are *primary and secondary questions*. Primary questions introduce topics or new areas. They can stand alone or out of context. "Where were you when the pain first started?" is an example. Secondary questions attempt to elicit more information, and they may be open or closed. Stewart and Cash (1978) refer to them as probing or follow-up questions which are used to get more complete or accurate data. They suggest that if the respondent has not completed an answer or is hesitant, the interviewer should remain silent while using nonverbal eye contact or head nodding. If the pause does not encourage the respondent to continue, probes such as "go on," can be used.

Mirror or summary questions reflect or summarize a series of questions and answers to make sure an accurate understanding has taken place. "Okay, let's see if I have this accurately. Your headaches always follow exposure to chocolate products?" is an example of a summary or mirror question.

The *reflective probing question* can also be used to help correct real or suspected inaccuracies. For example, the interviewer might say "Didn't you say you had four bouts with the flu?" These kinds of probes must be used carefully so that the respondent's integrity does not seem to be questioned.

By knowing a variety of questions and approaches, as well as being aware of the proper timing of questions, the interview can be personalized to meet the needs of the client and the practitioner (Stewart & Cash, 1978).

A nonjudgemental approach by the interviewer will encourage frank and free expression as well as emotional release. Sometimes it is necessary to show disapproval of behavior ("Ten packs a day??") but never of the client. Describing the data and the consequences rather than judging them are helpful techniques. The practitioner can make the observation "The available research data concludes that excessive smoking — and ten packs a day is in that category — is injurious to health," rather than the judgment "You are wrecking your life by such irresponsible smoking behavior."

As the interview progresses and trust is established, more direct, secondary questions can be asked. Once again, nonverbal clues provide helpful feedback. It is certainly appropriate to ask the client if he or she is satisfied with the progress of the interview, and an occasional summarizing of what has taken place is helpful. If the client does the summarizing, the practitioner has the opportunity to make sure that perceptions are mutually shared.

During the interview, health practitioners should monitor their own behavior. Are they listening or talking too much? What nonverbal signals are they sending to the client? Are they aware of prejudices they might have against the client such as size, color of skin, or manner? Are they using language clients understand without being patronizing?

Terminating the Interview

As the interview comes to a close, it is important for the client to know what other steps are required to solve the health problem and what resources are available for the solution. If other interviews or appointments are required, they should be clearly announced, agreed to by both parties, and clients should clearly understand why they are coming back. They should also be told the cost of all future interviews or procedures. It is important not to coerce the client into returning while making sure they have the necessary information to make that decision. As Enelow and Swisher (1972) state, "interviews build on each other." By giving the client information, the practitioner encourages client cooperation with the health care regimen. (Refer to our discussion of cooperation in chapter 1).

One last note. Before terminating the interview, all necessary paperwork should be rechecked to make sure that it is clear and accurate. Material which will be read by other members of the health care team should not violate the client's privacy. Additionally, it should be explained that others might see the record, if that is indeed the case.

Conventional medical records contain the client's history in six parts, usually in chronological sequence. Because this kind of record focuses on a simple illness or complaint, these records have been replaced in many health care settings by the problem-oriented record more frequently called the P.O.R. The goal of this method of record keeping is to develop a well-defined list of all the problems the client is experiencing with an effective data base. The P.O.R. (or P.O.M.R., Problem-oriented medical record) should be done several times in practice settings before being utilized on clients. Additionally, care must be taken in any record keeping not to diagnose or label the client prematurely without a complete data base.

Foley and Sharf (1981) have identified five interviewing techniques that are frequently overlooked in health care interviews: 1) putting the health care consumer at ease; 2) eliciting full and clear information; 3) maintaining control; 4) maintaining rapport; 5) bringing the interview to closure. The effective interviewer is aware of how to structure the interview, the goal to be achieved in the interview, the importance of adapting to the needs and feelings of the interviewee, and sharing feedback with the interviewee. (See Figure 3.2.)

The practitioner-client interview is the most important of health care interactions. The interview should be planned, and different questions and techniques should be applied as needed to each interview. The practitioner should be aware of the client's feelings, statements, and nonverbal behavior at all times. It is equally important for the interviewer to be aware of his or her own verbal and nonverbal behavior.

While the interview is of vital importance, there are many other situations in which communication takes place and interviewing is not the main objective. The overall communication behavior of the professional is often called "the bedside manner" and should be a product of the acquisition of good communication skills. As DiMatteo and Freidman (1982) indicate, it is a developed art. The professional must *learn* to communicate to the client that he or she is understood. A person who communicates effectively will monitor his or her own cues as well as those of the client and will consider social and psychological conditions such as culture and family experiences. The communication explanations in this book were written with these needs in mind.

In presenting the diagnosis to the client, Chenail et al. (1990) suggest that it is important to provide a context for medical findings and to give clients and families a framework in which they understand what is happening medically so that they can cooperate and share their medical information with others. As information about the illness or condition is conveyed to the patient and family, it is also important to read the client's nonverbal

Figure 3.2   The Five Categories of the Most Frequently Overlooked Interview Techniques Self Assessment Checklist

---

A. Beginning of the Interview:
Putting the patient at ease
1. Initiates a visit that puts the patient at ease.
2. Shows respect for patient by attending to needs of privacy and comfort.

B. Middle of the Interview:
Eliciting information
1. Uses open-ended questions to facilitate patient responses when appropriate.
2. Allows patient opportunity to explain story in own words without unnecessary interruptions.
3. Intervenes with appropriate responses when patient is unable to supply relevant information.
4. Rephrases or repeats question if needed to enhance understanding.
5. Clarifies areas of confusion or inconsistencies.
6. Inquires as to how well patient understands present illness.
7. Uses language appropriate to patient's age and background.
8. Aware of verbal habits (continuous okays, uh-huhs, noddings) that may be misunderstood by patient.

Maintaining control
9. Aware of pace of interview.
10. Uses periodic summaries.
11. Makes clear transitions from one step of the interview to another.
12. Interrupts unnecessary patient rambling to maintain focus.
13. Uses pauses to encourage patient response.

Maintaining Rapport
14. Maintains eye contact.
15. Uses nonverbal aspects (office seating arrangement, use of charts, body posture, facial expressions, touch) appropriately.
16. Allows opportunities for patient to express feelings about current illness and other problems.
17. Allows for sharing of feelings when appropriate.
18. Accepts patient's values in a nonjudgmental manner.
19. Sensitive to language or behavior that might arouse patient anxiety.
20. Explains the need for requesting certain data in order to reduce patient anxiety.
21. Deals with patient's expressed questions and concerns.
22. Deals with patient's nonverbally communicated concerns.

C. End of the Interview:
Bringing Closure
    1. Informs patient about next steps when appropriate.
    2. Allows patient opportunity to ask additional questions or add to the interview.
    3. Provides closing statements which facilitate a comfortable ending.

Reprinted with permission from Richard Foley and Barbara F. Sharf, "The Five Interviewing Techniques Most Frequently Overlooked by Primary Care Physicians." *Behavioral Medicine* II (1981): 30–31.

and verbal cues as well as to communicate support both nonverbally and verbally (Chenail, 1991; Ellis, Miller & Given, 1989).

Summary

This chapter addressed the client-practitioner relationship — a major focus of health communication research and literature.

Establishing a clear contract and understanding the dimensions of a therapeutic relationship are equally important. The components of such a relationship (empathy, trust, honesty, validation, and caring) were reviewed and listening skills were emphasized.

The health care interview, a major focus of health communication, was divided into planning, preparation (with a focus on time and space) and the development of the interaction. Procedures for asking questions, communicating findings, and terminating the interview were also presented.

up
munication
ealth Care

At Stanford University Hospital relationships in several of the operating rooms were becoming strained. Hostile and hurt feelings prevailed in an unsatisfactory work environment. Physicians, nurses and anesthesiologists were unhappy and needed to better understand each other's disciplines as they worked to deliver good health care. In an effort to solve these problems they formed a group to address and resolve problem issues (Mailhot and Slezak, 1983).

Despite technological increases and the availability of many of the resources needed to solve the basic needs of humankind, one essential ingredient often seems to be missing. Commentators on health care often note that we lack the ability to work together to solve problems ranging from health care in small settings to such global health-oriented issues as acid rain and the greenhouse effect. Lehman (1986) speculates that this is because of the hierarchical nature of health care systems.

In order to foster the collaboration necessary to solve complex problems in health care and other areas, individuals and organizations need to:

1. Learn how to set individual agendas aside in order to develop a common understanding of a problem.
2. Comprehend how that common understanding can be translated into action.
3. Develop the ability to coordinate people and their efforts within a structure that integrates and focuses energy rather than one which diffuses individual activities.
4. Foster the trust and the sharing of information that leads to the best decisions (Larson and LaFasto, 1989).

A small group is defined as three or more people whose behaviors exert a mutual and reciprocal influence on one another (Fisher, 1974). In this chapter small group issues in health care such as individual vs. group decision making, goals, social and task dimensions, roles, leadership, and climate will be reviewed. The last part of the chapter will focus on decision making and will summarize information on the most prevalent teams in contemporary health care — ethics committees, quality circles, and self-help groups.

Individual or Group Decision Making

It is not always simple to decide whether decisions would be best made and carried out by individuals or by groups. The surgical team is a good example of a contemporary task group. While this group needs to work carefully together, the surgeon is most often seen as the leader of the group and as the primary decision maker. With a small amount of time allocated for decision making, he or she has to make decisions and accept responsibilities. At the same time, the completion of a successful operation requires full participation by several people with various responsibilities in the decision-making process (Mailhot & Slezak, 1983).

In order to determine whether decisions should be made individually or consensually, groups or teams need to look at their tasks and goals in order to determine what kind of decision making is most appropriate. (Figure 4.1 provides information on individual and group decision making).

Figure 4.1

Criteria for Choosing a Group or Individual Problem-Solving Technique

Group Solutions Are Best	Individual Solutions Are Best
1. If there are many steps to the solution.	1. If there are just a few steps to the solution.
2. If there are many aspects to the problem.	2. If there are just a few aspects to the problem.
3. If the problem is impersonal.	3. If the problem is personal.
4. If the problem is of moderate difficullty.	4. If the problem is simple.
5. If several people are needed to provide the information to solve the problem.	5. If information to solve the problem can be provided by one person.
6. If the problem requires divisions of labor.	6. If the problem does not require divisions of labor.
7. If the problem requires several solutions.	7. If the problem requires just one solution.
8. If a great deal of time is required for solution of the problem.	8. If a small amount of time is required for solution of the problem.
9. If individuals have to assume a great deal of responsibility for the solution.	9. If individuals do not need to assume a great deal of responsibility.
10. If attitudes regarding the problem are going to be many and complex.	10. If attitudes toward the problem are going to be simple.
11. If it is likely group members will engage in task oriented behaviors.	11. If individuals will not be task oriented.

Goals, Climate and Tasks of the Group

Literature on small groups and leadership emphasizes the importance of mission statements or goals for a group (Larson & LaFasto, 1989; Bennis & Nanus, 1985). Goals must be clear, shared, and elevating or inspirational. In research conducted by Larson and LaFasto (1989), the clearest reason for team failure was deviation from the goal. They report that this lack of focus occurs because many group goals are complex and require a great deal of collaboration and concentration. Again, the operating team is a good example. Clarifying the goals of the team and *implementing* strategies to reach these goals were integral in the development of the group that was formed to solve the operating team's problems in the opening case study. The nurses had the unwritten goal of better communication with the physicians. The doctors felt that focusing on communication was "touchy-feely," and they wanted to concentrate instead on a discussion of specific tasks. It was only after these separate goals were discussed and clarified, that the team began solving its problems (Mailhot & Slezak, 1983).

In addition to goals and objectives, there are four elements that are important to all teams:

1. Clear roles and accountabilities;
2. An effective communication system;
3. The monitoring of individual performance with an effective feedback system which includes the ability to confront issues;
4. The need for objective and factual data for sound decision making (Larson and LaFasto, 1989).

Group climate, a subject of recent research, is also important for team development. *Climate* is the emotional tone of the group. It is the indicator of how comfortable group members are in their communication process. Supportive climate refers to working well together; it incorporates both feelings and structural features of teams that foster collaboration and trust. *Trust* includes the elements of honesty, openness, consistency and respect. Such trust is fragile; if broken, the climate of the team is compromised. It is trust that dominates the relationship of groups and teams that work well.

While groups are usually established for a particular purpose (such as providing health care to a client or serving as a management team for a health organization), every group has two built-in tasks: completing the group's assignment and maintaining the group's process and "social being." These tasks are often called the *task* and *social* dimensions. The social dimension is often overlooked in the planning of the project, but research indicates that this lack of planning is always a mistake. Humans are social beings, and they have many relationship needs. The expression of emotion is one example.

The *socio-emotional* climate which takes these needs into consideration is very important if the group is to function effectively. To determine the social, emotional, and/or psychological needs of individual members of the group, time has to be allocated within the group to explore these needs. The communication process is the vehicle by which members can do this. As team members understand the needs of others, behaviors interlock and members constrain their behavior while fitting into group patterns. As the group develops, certain members will play roles that help or hinder the socio-emotional dimensions of the group. The social aspect of groups is often called the *maintenance dimension*, because it helps maintain group member relationships.

In accomplishing the *task dimension*, which is usually the primary reason for the group's existence, groups are able to move efficiently only if they have *not* been negligent of the socio-emotional aspects. In this dimension, the group must clarify goals, assign responsibilities, and be accountable.

A communication climate which is *supportive* rather than *defensive* produces groups that fulfill the task and socio-emotional dimensions of the group more productively. According to Gibb (1961), supportive climates are characterized by being nonjudgmental, cooperatively independent, empathetic, and willing to experiment and be spontaneous. They reinforce participative planning and actions. Defensive climates are the opposite (see Figure 4.2). In health care, defensive climates are often characterized by blaming, time constraints, and a hierarchy that does not take individuals into consideration. They are judgmental, manipulative, emotionally neutral, and dogmatic. Unfortunately, most health related settings are defensive ones.

Figure 4.2

Supportive and Defensive Communication Climates

Supportive Climates	Defensive Climates
1. Description	1. Evaluation
2. Problem Orientation	2. Control
3. Spontaneity	3. Strategy
4. Empathy	4. Neutrality
5. Equality	5. Superiority
6. Provisionalism	6. Certainty

From Gibb, Jack R., "Defensive Communication." *Journal of Communication* 11, 1961, p. 147.

Roles

Roles in groups emerge around the social and task dimensions. A *role* is a position in an interlocking network. Generally, a role is defined in terms of the person occupying the role rather than by preordained actions. For example, physical therapists have roles to play in hospitals, but each therapist in the hospital enacts that role in a different way.

Roles are often categorized as *task, maintenance,* or *self-centered.* Role emergence takes place over time, and often group members play several roles. Roles can also change over the group's life span. *Task roles* involve such actions as initiating, giving information, seeking opinions, and being the person who elaborates and clarifies.

Maintenance roles involve the socio-emotional climate. Here group members support, harmonize, and give expression to relationship feelings.

Persons playing these roles sometimes act as "gatekeepers" who keep channels of communication open as tension relievers or compromisers. Examples of task and maintenance roles can be seen in Figure 4.3.

Other group members may play *self-centered* roles such as dominator or confessor. Self-centered roles often disrupt the effective functioning of the group and detract from group effectiveness. These should be discouraged in groups, while task and maintenance roles should be encouraged. While many roles are necessary for a fully functioning team, it is important to recognize that each member does not play all roles.

Figure 4.3   Group Roles

Group task roles help the group accomplish its jobs; group maintenance roles help the group solve its socio-emotional problems.

Group Task Role Examples

1. *Initiator-Contributor:* Contributes ideas and suggestions; proposes solutions, decisions, new ideas, or restates old ideas in novel ways.
2. *Information Seeker:* Asks for clarification in terms of the accuracy of comments; asks for information or facts relevant to accomplishing group tasks; suggests information if needed for decisions.
3. *Information Giver:* Offers facts or generalizations which may relate to personal experiences and are pertinent to the group task.
4. *Opinion Seeker:* Asks for clarification of group members' opinions; asks how group members feel.
5. *Opinion Giver:* States beliefs and opinions about suggestions made; indicates what the group's attitude should be.
6. *Elaborator-Clarifier:* Elaborates ideas and other contributions; offers rationales for suggestions; tries to deduce how an idea or suggestion would work if adopted by the group.
7. *Coordinator:* Clarifies relationships among information, opinions, and ideas; or suggests an integration of ideas.
8. *Diagnostician:* Indicates what the task oriented problems are.
9. *Orienter-Summarizer:* Summarizes interaction; points out departures from agreed upon goals; brings group back to the central issues; raises questions about the direction in which the group is headed.
10. *Energizer:* Prods the group to action.
11. *Procedure Developer:* Handles routine tasks such as seating arrangements, obtaining equipment, and handing out pertinent papers, etc.

12. *Secretary*: Keeps notes on the group's progress.

13. *Evaluator-Critic*: Analyzes the group's accomplishments; checks to see if consensus has been reached.

Maintenance Role Examples

1. *Supporter-Encourager*: Praises, agrees with, and accepts the contributions of others; offers warmth, solidarity and recognition.

2. *Harmonizer*: Reconciles and mediates differences; reduces tensions by giving group members a chance to explore their disagreements.

3. *Tension Reliever*: Jokes or, in some other way, reduces formality of interaction; relaxes the group members.

4. *Compromiser*: Offers to compromise when his or her own ideas are in conflict; admits own errors so as to maintain group cohesion.

5. *Gatekeeper*: Keeps communication channels open; facilitates interaction between some group members; blocks interaction between others.

6. *Feeling Expresser*: Makes explicit the feelings, moods and other relationships in the group; shares own feelings with others.

7. *Standard Setter*: Expresses standards in evaluating the group process and standards for the group to achieve.

8. *Follower*: Goes along with the movement of the group passively, accepting the ideas of others and sometimes serving as an audience for group interaction.

Self-Centered Role Examples

1. *Blocker*: Interferes with progress by rejecting ideas or taking the negative stand on any and all issues; refuses to cooperate.

2. *Aggressor*: Struggles for status by defining the status of others; boasts; criticizes.

3. *Deserter*: Withdraws in some way; remains indifferent, aloof, sometimes formal; daydreams; wanders from the subject; engages in irrelevant side conversations.

4. *Dominator*: Interrupts and embarks on long monologues; authoritative; tries to monopolize the group's time.

5. *Recognition Seeker*: Attempts to gain attention in an exaggerated manner; boasts about past accomplishments; relates irrelevant personal experiences, usually in an attempt to gain sympathy.

6. *Confessor*: Engages in irrelevant personal catharsis; uses the group to work out own mistakes and feelings.

7. *Playboy*: Displays a lack of involvement in the group through inappropriate humor, horseplay, or cynicism.

8. *Special-Interest Pleader*: Acts as the representative for another group; engages in irrelevant behavior.

Source: K. Benne and P. Sheats, "Functional Roles of Group Members." *Journal of Social Issues* 4 (1948): 41-49, with permission from the Society for the Psychological Study of Social Issues.

Leadership

Nowhere in America is hierarchy and status more evident than in health care. In most small groups, the physician is automatically the leader of an organized group through ascribed status. That is, he or she is made a leader by simple virtue of occupation. However, groups (such as health care teams with designated physician leaders) often develop informal leadership which bypasses physicians, if they are ineffective in the leadership role (Thornton, 1978).

In cases where this happens, the leadership role is usually assumed by the person who has provided the group with the most assistance in meeting its goals. While there are many kinds of leaders, it is important to recognize how each leader uses his or her power. For example, does the leader coerce others into making decisions or include others in the decision-making process? Gouran (1974) sees a leader as a person who uses his or her power to move or influence a group toward perceived goals through verbal and nonverbal communication.

There are three major leadership styles; autocratic, democratic, and *laissez-faire*. These three leadership styles vary in the degree of control they exert over the group and the decision-making process. Each of the three leadership styles has marked advantages and disadvantages for different group situations.

Autocratic leaders are very dominant and wield strong authority over group members. They tell group members what to do and how to do it. Sometimes they even watch the group members work to make sure they follow orders correctly. Autocratic leadership is probably the most common form of leadership in health care due to the high pressure climate and the control that doctors and administrators hold over others.

The major benefits of autocratic leadership are clear lines of authority, strong control, quick decisions, quick response time, and the ability of an expert leader to direct novice group members in complex or emergency tasks. However, the detriments of autocratic leadership often outweigh its advantages. Some of these disadvantages include the hindering of creativity by group members, dehumanization of group members, and lack of motivation by group members to abide by decisions. Autocratic leadership should only be used in emergency health care situations or where group members lack adequate knowledge of care methods. Unfortunately this model of leadership is often overused due in part to the military and religious antecedents of health care in which the autocratic models predominate.

Democratic leaders attempt to share authority appropriately with the group by eliciting information from all members and by asking for their participation in decision making. Often the democratic leader seeks consensus among group members. If consensus is unreachable, he or she seeks a majority vote.

Advantages of democratic leadership include active participation by all members, the sharing of expertise, the generation of a great deal of information, and the motivation and support of members. Disadvantages of the democratic style sometimes include the generation of extensive conflict when different perspectives are aired, the length of time required to hear members' opinions, the frustration of slow and labored decision making, and the potential for majority cliques to outvote and to manipulate smaller groups.

Democratic leadership is best used in complex problem-solving situations where a great deal of information and expertise is needed to make nonemergency decisions. For example, a group involved in long-range planning for an urban medical center should utilize democratic leadership in order to develop a workable model.

Laissez-faire leaders delegate authority to group members. Of all the leadership styles, laissez-faire is the most misunderstood and maligned. Often it is thought of as a "weak" form of leadership. In practice, however, laissez-faire leadership often requires the greatest strength of a leader. The leader must be confident enough in group members to allow them to make decisions on their own. The leader often provides the group with information and is available for problem solving but generally gives authority to the group for taking care of business.

Advantages of laissez-faire leadership include encouraging the growth and development of group members and the fostering of creative decision making. Disadvantages of laissez-faire leadership occur when the leader doesn't adequately prepare group members to work on their own or when group members are unable to handle the demands of the job and either take advantage of the situation or flounder in their performance. Laissez-faire leadership is best suited for well-trained, sophisticated, professional groups of people who can handle the task demands. An example of laissez-faire leadership might be an occupational therapy department of a community health organization where the department head assigns each therapist a case load and allows the therapist to decide the best means of treatment but remains available to help with problem solving. Laissez-faire leadership is also prominent in self-help groups not involving professionals.

No single leadership style is ever correct for all health care situations. The most competent leaders are able to adapt their leadership style to the particular group of people with whom they work and to the specific situations they confront. This is called *situational leadership*.

Lastly, one of the most important functions of the leader is to encourage group members to take responsibility for the group success. This can be accomplished, in part, by clarifying group responsibility and member roles to the satisfaction of group members during different phases of the group's existence.

As mentioned earlier, there can be separate task and socio-emotional leaders in groups although effective leaders are at least minimally efficient in both dimensions. Leadership skills can be learned, particularly through a study of communication processes.

Effective leaders must be able to inspire visions and goals for a group and to communicate intentions so that the group knows what the leader represents. They must also build and engender trust through reliability and constancy. Additionally, they should focus on competency, skill, and achieving success rather than failure. Effective leadership makes people feel that they are a significant part of a team or community (Bennis & Nanus, 1985).

Skills which can be developed and utilized by effective leaders are:

1. *Peer skills* — the ability to establish and maintain a network of contact with equals;

2. *Leadership skills* — the ability to deal with subordinates and all the complications that come with power, authority, and dependence;

3. *Conflict resolution skills* — the ability to mediate conflict and to handle disturbances under psychological stress;

4. *Information processing skills* — the ability to build networks, extract and validate information, and disseminate information effectively;

5. *Unstructured decision-making skills* — the ability to find problems and solutions when alternatives, information, and objectives are ambiguous;

6. *Resource allocation skills* — the ability to decide among alternative uses of time and other scarce organizational resources;

7. *Entrepreneurial skills* — the ability to take sensible risks and implement innovations;

8. *Introspection skills* — the ability to understand the effect leadership has on the organization (Mintzburg, 1973).

Many excellent books and articles have been written about leadership, although few of these discuss leadership in health care settings. One of the most impressive on general leadership is by James MacGregor Burns (1978). This book focuses on transformational leadership, a model that promotes leaders who create meanings and purposes for themselves and their subordinates. Burns suggests that an ideal leader enables followers to transcend daily affairs for higher purposes by helping them identify and carry out the primary goals and themes of the organization.

Conflict in Groups

The perspective group members have regarding conflict is important. If conflict is seen as constructive, the group will attempt to understand and manage it; if it is seen as destructive, it must be quickly resolved and controlled. The first approach allows for management, the second calls for dissolution.

Conflict in groups (or for that matter interpersonal conflict) is caused by many external and internal factors. Controversies over attempts to influence group members as well as attempts to influence a group's direction are often responsible for the conflict. In the process of creative conflict resolution, communication needs to be encouraged. Initially, it is important to decide who and what is in conflict. Conflict is observable and can be studied. For example, one can look at the interaction patterns of groups.

In defining a type of conflict, it is important to note if it is *affective*, (emotional) or *substantive* (intellectual opposition). It is, however, only in climates of mutual regard that conflict can be seen as issue oriented, which is the most useful kind of conflict. There are many strategies used by people facing conflict. They have been reviewed by Frost and Wilmot (1978) and much of the following material is abstracted from their book.

There are four primary conflict strategies people employ. *Avoidance* excludes active struggle. Those practicing this strategy sometimes refuse to talk, or they leave the conflict setting. The avoidance of conflict in initial stages is common in health organizations where the benefits of conflict are not recognized. Changing the subject is a common avoidance tactic. *Escalation* can include such tactics as labeling, increasing the intensity of the struggle, and yelling or violence. It can also include a purposeful expansion of the issue beyond its legitimate limits. Coalition formation can also cause escalation. This occurs when several members of a group band together — a group of radiation therapists who want their hours changed, for example. *Reduction* is a conflict strategy designed to lessen the conflict before it has been allowed to develop. Again, if one's perspective is that conflict can be healthy and creative for a group, this is not always an effective technique since it squelches needs and issues that must surface before the problem can be understood and resolved. A nurse who tells his or her colleagues that a breakdown in communication is not important is using a reduction technique. *Maintenance*, the last conflict strategy, keeps the conflict at a tension level which is manageable to each of the combatants. Maintenance tactics are designed to equalize the power of the participants or to gain symmetry. An example of the maintenance technique is the quid pro quo in which each party gets something for something. Professional schools, hospitals, and other health care settings need to train their employees to recognize and apply useful and appropriate conflict strategies not only to solve problems but also to reduce tension.

Group conflict becomes complicated when different members use diverse conflict strategies and the strategies are accompanied by emotions such as anger. Anger is usually the vehicle by which conflict is expressed in groups. While it can sap energy from groups, it can also galvanize conflict resolution. In order to be used in a positive way, anger needs to be recognized as a legitimate emotion which will not destroy the group or its members if used ethically. Anger is particularly difficult to deal with in hierarchical settings (such as health care) where power resides at the top. Subordinates fear expressing anger because of unequal power, yet suppressing anger may be more detrimental to the group than expressing this emotion. As hospitals and private offices deal with such problems as nurse retention, it is important to recognize the anger that nurses have regarding their place in the health care hierarchy. Dealing with this anger would be cost efficient for these organizations.

Conflict can be both productive and destructive for groups. The destructive aspects of conflict are usually emphasized more than the positive aspects. Often people fail to recognize the constructive opportunities afforded by group conflict. For example, conflict is crucial if the group is to avoid *group think*, where members go along with what they perceive to be the group's decision regardless of their own judgment. Conflict will allow group members to see different aspects of a problem and can provide the opportunity for creative problem solving.

There are six primary benefits of group conflict that people normally do not consider.

1. Conflict acts as a kind of smoke detector for the group by often helping members to identify larger underlying problems that should be addressed by the group.

2. Conflict acts as a safety valve for the group by allowing the release of tension and anger.

3. Conflict encourages interaction and involvement of group members in discussing issues of concern.

4. Conflict promotes creative behavior by group members by encouraging the search for solutions to problems.

5. Conflict promotes the sharing of relevant information among group members by encouraging the voicing of disparate ideas.

6. Conflict tests the strength of group members' ideas and their potential solutions under fire by arguing the relative merits of proposed ideas and solutions.

One of the most effective techniques for looking at anger, power, and thus conflict in small groups is *process observation*. As discussed in chapter 2, there are two aspects of each communicative act: content and relationship. The content level focuses on how members of the group present the basic information in the message. The relationship level refers to the feelings expressed, particularly through nonverbal channels. *Process observation* provides the group with a means of evaluating group communication by having an observer assess the group at both content and relationship levels. The observer can be someone who has no ties to the group, or a group member can be trained for this function. This observer reports back to the group at the end of the session on what he or she saw happening within the group. Process observers need some training in observation techniques; at the minimal level, they need to understand what the group wants from the observation.

Sometimes check lists or interaction analysis schemes are used for the observation. Most important, the processor must be nonevaluative and be able to describe what he or she saw. Material presented to the group in a fair manner can often be the starting point for effective discussion. The role of the process observer needs to be clearly negotiated and understood by all the group members before process observation begins. The process observer and/or a third-party negotiator, who seeks to solve the conflict as well as to observe it, can be separate or one and the same. However, a person unskilled in arbitration should not undertake to solve a group's problem. Additionally, while members of the group can learn to take the observer's role, they cannot effectively act as negotiators of a conflict in which they participate.

The negotiator has many strategies available for helping the group. First, he or she can assist the group in clarifying and implementing its goals as well as by providing a safe atmosphere within the group for effective feedback. The negotiator helps to equalize power within the group. Techniques such as role reversal can sometimes be effective. Group members can also be assisted in prioritizing and dealing with problems.

In attempting to come to some form of conflict resolution, group members or the negotiator must think of strategies. Should everyone who is part of the conflict win in some way or should there be a *win-lose* outcome? It is even possible to structure a conflict situation in which everyone loses or everyone wins (Fisher, 1974).

Understanding the structure of the conflict helps determine the solutions. It also makes clear that parties to the conflict must have an equal say in determining the choices and the payoffs if the solution is going to be effective and permanent. It is important to develop a climate of openness, honest acceptance, and cohesiveness for conflict resolution. Getting to the roots of the conflict in a group can be important. Ultimately, members should feel good about their personal contribution to a group. This feeling can take place in an atmosphere of debate or strong feelings as long as individual differences are respected.

Ethical conflict behaviors are also important to discuss. In conflict situations, arguing the specific issue at hand is an important fair-fighting technique. In a supportive group atmosphere, violence, character attacks, and "dirty-fighting" techniques should be avoided. On the positive side, it is important to construct reasonable arguments rather than emotional, unsubstantiated positions. Lastly, a "gamesman," win-at-all-costs mentality can be avoided by being open to the ideas of others for a *mutual-win* solution. Conflict is rarely a *zero-sum* game where one person must win at the expense of others.

Dealing with conflict in health care or other settings is time consuming, but it can be beneficial to the group if conducted ethically. Participants need to be educated about how to handle conflict well. We suggest that the time taken to educate individuals in effective conflict communication skills will save money and be energy efficient.

Decision Making in Groups

As groups become more prominent in health care, effective decision making and problem solving is important. There are many models for understanding the process of making group decisions. It is important to remember that decision making is not always problem solving. For example, a decision by a group to disband their work fifteen minutes early on a Friday afternoon is not dealing with a problem! Decisions have to do with the outcome of group interaction. A *decision* is the choice made by group members from the available alternative proposals. A group can sometimes reach a decision by consensus. *Consensus* has many meanings. It can imply unanimous agreement, the will of the majority, or implicit agreement. For practical purposes, it means a commitment to the decision reached.

Research on groups indicates that consensual decision making is desirable in order to encourage all group members to own and fully implement decisions (Ducanis & Golin, 1979; Eichhorn, 1974; Thornton, 1978).

Groups, as well as individuals, go through processes or phases to reach their decisions though there is no one proven way that this takes place. In Fisher's decision emergence scheme (1974), ideas pass through the *orientation phase* where members socialize, orient themselves to the issues, and relieve primary tension. In the *conflict phase*, there is a dispute and ideas are tested while coalitions develop. In the *emergence phase* there is much ambiguity in the group as members try to arrive at the "best" decision. This third and crucial stage marks the beginning of the eventual outcome of the group. In the *reinforcement phase* unity of opinion usually pervades as courses for group action are prescribed.

Decision making is the first step in any problem-solving process. *Problem solving* involves using communication techniques to both make decisions as well as to carry out decisions. There may be several decisions made and implemented in the course of problem solving.

Problem-solving techniques are important for health care groups and for health care professionals. Some problems are best suited to group solution, while others are best suited to individual solution, as discussed earlier in this chapter.

The problem solver must first decide what constitutes a problem. For example, the hospital administrator must decide if tardiness of employees in the spring is due to a temporary change in the weather or if it is indicative of an overall more serious pattern for the institution. A problem exists for an individual when he or she becomes aware of the obstacle or obstacles to obtaining a goal. Problems can involve familiar or unfamiliar material as well as subjective or objective material.

Problem solving is both an ability and a process. A problem-solving action-oriented scheme has been developed by Thornton and is included in chapter 8 in this book. While oriented to ethics, it can be utilized in all decision making, whether or not decisions have a moral component.

There are many methods to help groups develop consensus. The Delphi technique involves questioning, planning and canvassing experts. The Nominal Group technique requires a trained facilitator and a group which responds in writing to the facilitator's questions. There are also consensus developing conferences designed to help diverse members achieve general agreement. Focus groups are sometimes utilized in health care for research purposes. Researchers seek in-depth discussions of topic areas necessary for future research and planning. Information on using these techniques can be found in Cline (1990).

Brainstorming

One of the successful techniques for decision making that does not involve a trained facilitator or much planning is brainstorming. It is a useful way to generate ideas and to avoid polarized yes-no answers to problem-solving issues. *Brainstorming* encourages unique and creative solutions to problems. When brainstorming, it is important to get the group to abide by the following rules:

1. Anything goes. Get your ideas on paper. Sometimes wild ideas are the best ones or can be combined with other ideas for innovative solutions.
2. Don't be evaluative as the ideas are being presented. Just listen!
3. Think of as many ideas as you can. Allow the session to go on as long as possible. Brainstorming doesn't work as well when members have to rush to another meeting! However, if you are limited by time, make the deadlines clear to group members.
4. Record all ideas so that everyone can see them. Newsprint or blackboards are helpful.
5. Take a break between brainstorming and evaluating. When evaluation does take place be positive, fair, and go slowly toward your solution.

Because brainstorming starts out as nonevaluative, it can prevent many of the difficulties that occur when groups form judgements of individuals or ideas too early in the group decision-making process.

Much of our work and play in today's world takes place in cooperative effort with others. An understanding of what makes people work well together is vital in order to be an effective group member. Continued research on groups is also important in order to help us identify and understand the group communication process. In the following sections, we will use case studies as examples of groups in health care including the health team, the ethics committee, quality circles, and the self-help group.

Health Teams and Group Communication

Dr. G. S. Edwards is a well-known oncologist determined to make the detection and treatment of cancer bearable and humane. She has developed an effective team approach, utilizing a receptionist who has been trained in counseling and three nurses trained in oncology.

The doctor's office serves as the hub of a wheel, with the objective of including the family and the patient in all aspects of treatment. The receptionist and chemotherapy room are within steps of Dr. Edwards who is almost instantly available for consultation if problems arise. The nurses and the receptionist-counselor are trained by the doctor in communication, cancer, and chemotherapy. These members of the team often answer initial client questions or serve as intermediaries if the doctor is out of the office. Clients calling the office are always able to talk to a member of the oncology team. Quite often, Dr.

Edwards will interrupt whatever she is doing to take these phone calls. As much as possible, the same staff sees the client on each visit.

The examining room is in the doctor's cheerful office. Family members are encouraged to accompany the client and stay in the room with the curtain separating them from the doctor and the client during the examination, unless the client directs otherwise. Note taking is common. Often, hours are spent educating the family regarding the various treatment alternatives. The theory utilized is that well-educated clients and family members can be capable participants in the decision-making and treatment phases. Families are also taught to become active in the treatment process. If shots are required, they learn to give these shots in Dr. Edwards' arm, which psychologically removes much of the threat of this procedure. During the twenty-four hours after the first treatment, the doctor often makes a house call to check on both client and family. Later, during treatment, the receptionist-counselor might also visit the client in home or hospital settings.

The members of the oncology team are chosen carefully. The receptionist-counselor has conducted support groups and worked in other health care settings. The nurses were carefully picked for their concern about clients, their relaxed manner, and their ability to communicate. The team members report that they like each other and feel trust in their professional relationships. Meetings are held on a daily basis and the doctor listens carefully as well as participates. She is quite aware that the client provides different kinds of information to each team member, and it is during the meetings that all the information is integrated and put to use for the client's benefit.

Family members also report feeling part of the extended family effort. They credit the initial time spent educating them regarding the illness as reassuring during the whole treatment. Additionally, being involved gives them something to do at a time when most of them are feeling useless and frustrated. They also note that neither they nor the client have to call the doctor often during the treatment process because of the adequate preparation.

Dr. Edwards' clients do not follow the usual national pattern where large numbers of people drop out of chemotherapy during the treatments. In addition, they report reduced side effects. The clients credit open communication and the team process with giving them needed support and more bearable treatments.

Dr. Edwards is candid about the advantages of the team system. The initial time spent with the client and the family prevents excessive phone calls to her. The fully functioning team shares the pressure and allows her to supervise and be more aware of the overall client regimen and profile. It also frees her to keep up-to-date professionally and to work with her colleagues. She particularly stresses that the time taken with clients by team members induces client cooperation during the treatment regime, which in turn reduces morbidity and raises the response rate to the treatment because of better patient toleration. Clearly, this physician's office operates as an effective health-related small group.

The advantages and disadvantages of team care such as this will be discussed in the following pages.

Health care team generally refers to a group of people, often from different disciplines, who work collaboratively with the specific purpose of delivering better care to clients. Beckhard (1972) states that a team exists when tasks require interdependence of persons with different technical skills.

The experiences of diverse groups and teams are reported in the literature. Teams in psychiatric settings have been designed to improve patient treatment plans (Toseland, Palmer-Geneles & Champman, 1986) and to improve patients' interpersonal skills (Pelletier, 1983). Ward treatment teams are reported in Great Britain (Humphris, 1988) and executive interdisciplinary management teams which focus on the smooth running of a department or organization related to health care are being developed (Farley & Stoner, 1989).

Occupational therapy teams, rehabilitation teams, and primary care nursing teams are also seen as efficient and collaborative ways to deal with client problems (Moulder, Staal, & Grant, 1988). For example, McManus (1989) reports on third world ophthalmic teams which assist in preventing or assisting with difficult eye problems. Teams also exist for health professionals who support each other in an attempt to deliver care to persons with AIDS (Bolle, 1989).

Case management is a current model used by many health care teams. While the case management model is not always considered collaborative, it generally consists of multidisciplinary involvement. Case management, often advocated as the ideal model of patient care by nurses, utilizes both clinical expertise with a business approach to managing care. The case manager (usually a nurse) serves as the team leader, functioning as a clinical expert and coordinator of care. He or she collaborates with other primary care givers and service providers (Salmond, 1990; Humphris, 1988).

The operating room dilemma cited in the case study at the beginning of this chapter illustrates communication problems common to many small groups. In this case, a collaborative team was established by the operating room staff to bridge the communication and task-related problems between doctors and nurses. A problem-oriented focus improved communication, and a documentation of problems and problem-solving techniques helped these professionals (Mailhot & Slezak, 1983).

The growing body of literature on health care teams indicates that client and professional satisfaction grows when health care teams function successfully. When they do not, problems include conflict, misunderstanding of roles, miscommunication, lack of time, and hierarchical differences (Thornton, et al, 1980).

The Ethics Committee

A sixty-two-year-old woman was hospitalized for gallbladder surgery. There were numerous complications after the operation, and she did not recover. After ten days she lapsed into a coma. The doctors gave the family choices regarding whether the patient should remain on the respirator and whether a medication which would prevent pneumonia should be continued. The family was divided about what should be done. They decided to consult an ethics committee.

In the last ten years, this nation has seen the development of a collaborative effort in health care known as the ethics committee. An *Ethics Committee* is a group of health care providers and sometimes consumers who focus on the moral issues of health care in a work setting. These committees are now estimated to exist in 60 percent of American hospitals (Cohen, 1988). One of the reasons for their existence is to assist families and health care providers in solving such problems as the one presented here.

Ethics committees are often organized by the hospital administration; their membership consists of physicians, representatives from the nursing staff, social workers, and sometimes administrators and clergy. Less frequently, community representatives, family members and sometimes an ethicist are included. The purpose of an ethics committee is to assist health care practitioners and families in making difficult moral decisions such as the case involving the comatose patient. In addition to case consultation, the functions of committees are to educate and formulate policy on such matters as DNR orders (do not resuscitate) and neonatal unit procedures (Ross, 1986; Cranford & Doudera, 1984).

The growing body of literature on ethics committees indicates that when organized and operated effectively, they are an asset to professionals, families, patients, and the institution. Corrine Bayley (1986) one of the national leaders of the ethics committee movement, speaks about the need to deal with the committee's interpersonal relationships if committees are to move forward with their functions of education, policy making, and case review. She suggests that an understanding of group dynamics enables committees to function more effectively.

The communication problems of ethics committees, particularly those regarding group interaction, are similar to those of the health care team with one added dimension: dealing with different views of morality. Ethics committees are sometimes criticized for diluting decision-making authority and for ignoring the viewpoints of patients and families in their deliberations. Committees often invite consultants such as philosophers or other specialists in the field of bioethics to assist them. In the view of the authors of this text, communication specialists, with some understanding of the moral dimensions of human behavior, can be especially helpful to ethics committees as consultants.

Quality Circles

In a mental unit in North Warwickshire, England there were twenty permanent residents (twelve woman and eight men) who were both hyperactive and physically handicapped. Each day these twenty patients had to be bathed, dressed, and fed by a staff of four in one hour and fifteen minutes in a poorly equipped area. In addition to the shortage of staff and of time, the unit was being criticized for poor service, staff performance and delivery of care. A frustrated administration decided to adopt the quality circle concept. After several meetings, the staff defined and solved what seemed to be an intractable problem. Quality circles have great potential for health care (Johnson & Clarke, 1984).

A *quality circle* is defined as a small group (usually ten or twelve people) from a specific part of an organization who voluntarily meet to identify and work on specific short-term problems identified either by them or the administration (Stohl, 1986). The QC concept assumes that those who *do* the job, regardless of their place on the hierarchy, *know* the job and therefore can solve identified problems closest to them.

The goal of a quality circle is to provide means for staff to become genuinely involved with the organizational policies that affect them and to give people throughout the organization a chance to develop their skills as well as to solve specific organizational problems. Supporters of this concept contend that QCs also can generate tangible financial benefits when they identify and solve problems in a timely manner (Robson, 1984).

The quality circle concept, adapted from the Japanese, has been slow to make its way into the health care system, although it is a prominent work technique in manufacturing and business. In 1985 it was estimated that over 90 percent of the Fortune 500 companies had implemented the quality circle concept (Lawler & Mohrman, 1985). Robson (1984) contends that health care organizations can learn a valuable lesson from industry if they realize that in the future they must rely on their staff at all levels to help resolve the increasingly complicated issues of health care. The slow growth of quality circles in health settings is attributed to the fact that the concept is participative and health care has commonly leaned toward more centralized status quo and hierarchical forms of management (Lehman, 1986).

Research on quality circles indicates that once they are well-received by workers and by management, they improve morale, increase loyalty, foster teamwork, and improve productivity and quality of service. Additionally, they reduce absenteeism, tardiness, accidents, and lost time and service (Thompson, 1982). While not designed to make radical organizational change, these groups modify the communication patterns and the culture of an organization (Stohl, 1986).

The quality circle concept supports the rationale for small group decision making which states that in effective consensual decision making, involved parties take ownership of the decision and provide the support that allows decisions to be implemented (Tinello-Biddle, 1986).

The few published reports on quality circles in health care are generally favorable. However, problems inherent in other health care groups are reported. A prime difficulty is scheduling time for the team members to meet. When the team does not meet frequently, frustration and disappointment occur and the momentum and enthusiasm of the team is diminished. The importance of employing good communication and decision-making techniques in these groups is consistently discussed by writers on the subject. Critics also contend that workers involved in quality circles sometimes adopt a management perspective which can be detrimental to their independence within an organization (Stohl, 1987).

Self-Help Groups

David just found out he had acquired immunodeficiency syndrome (AIDS). He was twenty-seven and had not told his parents he was gay. No one suspected his diagnosis. He felt he needed to talk to other persons with AIDS about family and treatment dilemmas. A friend referred him to an AIDS support group.

In the late 1970s, it was estimated that between 15 and 20 million people were involved in 500,000 self-help groups (Arntson & Droge, 1987). Alcoholics Anonymous pioneered this development. Groups giving support to cancer patients (Heiney & Wells, 1989) as well as to persons with AIDS (Ribble, 1989) are examples of people who organize around a particular need. These organizations are often started by persons who want to find others who share the same problem. Members are given a chance to report case histories and personal thoughts and to develop social support (Albrecht & Adeleman, 1987). *Social support* is a process that helps distressed individuals through the anxiety and uncertainty of difficult life events. Self-help groups which provide social support are sometimes run by nonprofessionals, although persons with expertise are usually part of the start-up process (Heiney & Wells, 1989). Alternatively, therapeutic groups in such settings as rehabilitation and psychiatry utilize professionals throughout the group process, although the focus is still on self-help.

Self-help groups give members a reason to talk. There is a sanctioned time and place for support and an important informal opportunity for contact outside the formal meeting structure. A study of groups composed of epileptics indicated the importance of stories in the self-help groups, so that members realize commonalities. Group members rid themselves of the stigma of their illness or problem by giving advice and helping others (Arnston & Droge, 1987).

These groups sometimes suffer from a lack of organization. Like many small groups, there is sometimes a lack of agreement about goals and processes. Self-help clearinghouses as well as popular columns in magazines and newspapers are helpful to those wanting to research, consult, or start self-help groups (Madara, 1987).

An increasing emphasis is being placed on support groups for professionals who work in highly stressful settings. Reporting on social support for hospice teams, Richman (1989, p. 8) acknowledges the importance of six kinds of support.

1. *Listening*: actively listen without giving advice or making judgments; share the joys of success as well as the frustration of failure.

2. *Technical appreciation*: acknowledge when a good piece of work has been accomplished.

3. *Technical challenge*: be knowledgeable about an individual's work and challenge, stretch, and encourage the individual to achieve more and to be more creative and excited about her or his work.

4. *Emotional support*: support individuals during an emotionally difficult time without necessarily agreeing with them.

5. *Emotional challenge*: challenge an individual to do her or his best to overcome obstacles and fulfill goals.

6. *Sharing social reality*: verify perceptions of the social context and reveal similar priorities, values, and perspectives in order to serve as a reality touchstone

Whether the group is organized for clients or for professionals, it is increasingly clear that self-help or support groups are an important part of health care.

Focus Groups in Health Care

Sex education was becoming a highly volatile issue in a midwestern school district. Liberal and conservative groups were arguing about whether such programs should exist and, if so, how they should be organized.

While the new school superintendent felt strongly that such programs were an important part of education, she also believed that such educational offerings should incorporate the feelings and ideas of both parents and students. She instructed her assistant to explore the focus group concept.

Focus groups, sometimes called exploratory groups, are a qualitative research tool increasingly popular with marketing experts in health care and other fields. They are used to obtain insights into perceptions, language, beliefs, values, and attitudes of target groups. For example, a focus group might be convened to analyze what teenagers know about herpes in order to design a campaign to prevent such diseases. Such groups usually consist of eight to ten participants and are run by a qualified moderator. The moderator or discussion leader makes sure certain areas are covered through the skillful use of a protocol or a plan that allows open discussion. It is particularly important that the focus group moderator be well-trained and have some training in small group dynamics (U.S. Dept. of Health & Human Services, 1989). Transcripts of the groups' deliberations should be analyzed by group specialists.

Focus groups are sometimes criticized for being too subjective and too preliminary (Calder, 1977; Greenbaum, 1989) especially when the results are overgeneralized. However, advocates of such groups argue that they are justified when more controlled scientific techniques cannot be utilized (Calder, 1977). It is also argued that focus groups are especially useful in the concept stages of developing a project (Calder, 1977; U.S. Dept. of Health & Human Services, 1989).

The health communication and education fields are increasingly utilizing focus groups (U.S. Dept. of Health & Human Services, 1989). One such program convened focus groups to find a logo for a heart disease program while a second series of focus groups investigated the knowledge and attitudes of white, Black and Hispanic men and women regarding breast cancer (NCI, 1984). Other health-related focus groups have involved contraception and pregnancy (Kisker, 1985), smoking prevention (Heimann, Hanson & Peregoy, 1985), and marketing research (Basch, 1987).

AIDS marketing and research has utilized focus groups to analyze college students' behavior (Cline & Freeman, 1988) and Black viewpoints (Herscher, 1991). In the latter study, African American women infected with the AIDS virus or women who were caregivers to those with AIDS provided information for the redesign of an educational campaign that in prior versions had been criticized as being highly offensive to Blacks.

Focus groups have become widely used in health care, but programs utilizing such groups should be well-designed. The preliminary findings of such groups should be subject to further program enhancement and design. Certainly, the future of such groups should be of interest to health communication specialists.

In summary, small groups are an important part of health care. They are particularly useful if consensual — when the group agrees with the results of the decision making. Cline (1990) analyzes such groups and also provides an in-depth discussion of consensual techniques such as the Delphi technique and Nominal Group process which assist in this consensual decision making.

Health teams, quality circles, self-help and focus groups are just a few examples of the types of groups useful for health care. While it is important that more research be done on each of these models so that we can understand their particular problems and needs, there is much we already know about small groups that can be used to make them more effective in specific settings.

Special Problems for Health Care Providers in Group Settings

As can be seen from the previous discussion of small groups, interacting with others is complex. This complexity increases in health care settings where strong emotions, status differences, and time pressures interact.

Dealing with psychosocial issues is not easy, as indicated by the Stanford Hospital example where nurses wanted to deal with feelings and communication while physicians wanted to work on problem solving. Establishing goals and objectives for groups which are both task and maintenance based enables the needs of diverse groups and individuals to be fulfilled.

Additionally, it is important to consider barriers to communication. Group members often have different perceptions of health and how it should be achieved. Some health training institutions emphasize service while others highlight research. The two orientations can provide much conflict unless both are valued by the group and the administration.

Communication in groups is also affected by the information flow regarding knowledge about another's field. Because of the hierarchical status of health care, the information received by group members is influenced by their relative status within the organization. The articulation of roles is primarily a result of accommodating the lower status professions to those of high status. This freezing of status limits the possibilities of reexamining the roles and realigning the boundaries of the different fields in order to deliver effective health care (Nagi, 1975).

Team literature has recently focused on decision making and conflict management. Sources regarding groups in health care stress the importance of members spending time with each other in order to better understand each other so that tasks can be accomplished effectively. This provides a double-bind for providers who feel that their time should be spent in actual care giving rather than in solving problems.

The problems of turf management and overlapping roles are also difficult. Innovative teams and groups have learned to conduct rounds together, integrate chart notes, and meet weekly in order to avoid these problems.

After three years of research on health teams, Thornton, McCoy and Baldwin (1980) found that most team energy is spent trying to manage relationships within the teams. In order to accomplish necessary tasks, energy needs to be balanced between structure, content, and process. Team training is vitally important in order for effective functioning to take place whether the group is a health team, an ethics committee, or a self-help group.

Whatever the problems of health teams and groups, they have become important to client care. Health and medical literature abound with references. In addition, health providers, regardless of their position, are beginning to demand input into client care and the team or group is a vehicle for this input.

Hidden barriers to group and team building are described by Palleschi and Heim (1980). Barriers refer to norms which are often unwritten rules. Members are punished for violating norms or rewarded for adhering to them. In order to avoid these barriers, the following should happen:

1. Group members should have the same level and type of knowledge about the problem. This does not mean that they need the same

discipline knowledge, but they should share information about the problem the team is addressing. Jargon of the various disciplines can impede such knowledge flow and build "in" and "out" groups in the team setting.

2. Sharing territory is important to effective group functioning. Meetings should be held in neutral territory which does not hinder the flow of information.

3. The stature of members during meetings needs to be as equal as possible in order for knowledge sharing to be open. Round tables promote information flow as does a room that is physically comfortable and has pleasant surroundings.

4. The opportunities to communicate among participants needs to be equal. Group networks need to be open and not operate exclusively through just one member. It is helpful for communication purposes if members are often in proximity to each other or at least have a common gathering place to share information.

Summary

In this chapter the importance of small groups in the health care setting was discussed. The goals and climates of the group were emphasized, as was the importance of acknowledging both the task and maintenance functions. This theme, in fact, pervades the chapter. Leadership, conflict resolution, and role negotiation are intertwined with an understanding of both the task (or content) and maintenance (or psychosocial) concerns. Finally, some special groups in health care including ethics committees, quality circles, self-help groups, and focus groups were discussed.

CHAPTER
5

Organizational Communication in Health Care

There was trouble at Glenview County Hospital. The morale of hospital employees was at an all time low. Several key staff members had tendered their resignations, and there was a rumor circulating among the hospital staff that widespread administrative changes and restructuring were in the offing. The low morale, which caused poor staff attitudes and internal squabbles, was affecting the quality of health care. Bob Wilson, the chief administrator of the hospital was worried. He didn't know what was going on at the hospital nor what he should do about it.

Bob Wilson had been hired three months ago by his predecessor, Frank Hyatt, who retired after fourteen years with the hospital. Before coming to Glenview, Bob had been the assistant administrator at a nearby hospital for a little less than two years. Prior to that, he had received *a master's degree in health administration from the state university. Neither his past employment nor his education had prepared him for the low morale situation at Glenview.*

Bob decided to bring in his two assistant administrators to discuss the morale situation and find out what was at the root of the problem. They both corroborated the fact that there was a problem and, in fact, told Bob that they both had heard from several "reliable sources" about the upcoming administrative layoffs. The more Bob denied the layoffs, the more suspicious the assistant administrators became. They wanted to know why he couldn't confide in them and tell them what was "really" going on. Eventually they began to assume that they were both potential victims of the administrative restructuring they were certain was being planned.

Bob was even more concerned about the morale situation after talking to his assistants. It seemed that no matter what he did, the people working for him were becoming more and more paranoid. He gave Frank Hyatt a call and asked if Frank had any idea what was going on at the hospital. Frank said he had never encountered a serious morale problem in all his years as an administrator at Glenview. In fact, he had always felt that morale at the hospital was excellent, like a big happy family. This didn't make Bob feel any better about the situation.

Bob decided to call in one of his former professors from the university who was an expert in organizational behavior as an external consultant to help solve the morale problem. The consultant began his work by interviewing different members of the hospital staff. Again and again he heard the same story; they believed the new hospital administrator was planning a major administrative reorganization including massive layoffs. When asked where they had heard of this reorganization several different names were mentioned. One name, however, was identified as a source of information by almost everyone: Horace Jackson, a hospital janitor.

Horace was sixty-four years old and had been with the hospital for more than thirty years. He was well-liked within the organization, and, in fact, spent a good deal of his time each day wheeling a large plastic trash container around the hospital and visiting with members of each hospital department. When the consultant interviewed Horace, he claimed he hadn't heard of any layoffs. The consultant recognized the contradictions between the report he received from Horace and those he had received from other members of the hospital staff and realized that Horace was probably the initial source of the rumor about layoffs.

When the consultant informed Bob Wilson of what he had found, Bob reacted angrily and wanted to fire Horace. The consultant warned against hasty action and told Bob that firing Horace would only serve to confirm the false rumor about layoffs. If Horace, who had been with the hospital for thirty years, was expendable, then the hospital staff would really be convinced the rumor was true. Instead, the consultant suggested that Bob recognize that Horace was an informal leader in the organization and could be nurtured as an organizational ally rather than an enemy.

Bob called Frank Hyatt again and asked what he knew about Horace Jackson. Frank replied that Horace was one of his most trusted employees — that he had taken special care of Horace. He had invited him into his office every once in a while and asked him how things were going. Horace provided Frank with information about what was happening behind the scenes at the hospital. Frank said he usually sought advice from Horace about problems at the hospital and was generally given good advice. Every Christmas Frank made sure to give Horace a bottle of scotch as a present. Bob began to realize how important an individual Horace was in the hospital. He recalled how curt he had been when Horace had dropped by his office during his first week and asked if he needed any help. Bob was busy with some details and had offhandedly dismissed Horace's offer of help. Bob realized that Horace had probably been insulted and had retaliated by starting the rumor about hospital layoffs.

Bob followed the consultant's advice and began to nurture his relationship with Horace. He invited Horace to have lunch with him at the hospital cafeteria and asked for the janitor's advice about improving hospital morale. He shared some of his ideas about improving the quality of health care at the hospital with Horace. Over the next month Bob encouraged Horace to drop by his office to discuss any problems or ideas Horace had. Over this same time period, the rumor about layoffs began to subside and morale began to improve. Horace was now sending new information through the organization about what an excellent administrator Bob Wilson was!

In this case history, much of the hospital's informal communication was working against the goals of the organization. To solve the morale problems in the organization the hospital administrator had to redirect organizational communication. In this chapter we will explore the different ways communication affects organizational activities. We will see how important communication is in effective health care organizations.

Human beings organize their activities with one another to accomplish complex tasks. As the modern world has grown more and more complex, the need for organized human activities has grown, as evidenced by the great abundance of organizations that affect our lives. Some of the most important organizations in our lives are health care organizations.

The health care organization is the primary setting for health care practice. Hospitals, medical centers, health maintenance organizations, clinics, nursing homes, and convalescent centers have developed as centers for health care delivery in the modern world. Human communication in these health care organizations enables health professionals, health care support staff, and clients to coordinate their activities to accomplish health care goals.

Communication in organizations enables members to share important information about the goals, structures, problems, and strategies of the organization. Yet ineffective communication can block the fulfillment of organizational goals and further complicate the health care delivery system by distorting information, blocking the exchange of important messages, and alienating health care workers from one another. In this chapter we will examine the development of effective communication in health care organizations.

Message Flow in Health Care Organizations

Message flow in organizations has traditionally been described in terms of *formal organizational structure*. The formal structure of an organization follows the *organizational chart*, which maps the prescribed hierarchy of power relationships that exist within an organization. Depending on the job titles and job descriptions people have within their organizations, certain formal relationships between organization members are prescribed in the performance of their job responsibilities. For example, the people to whom you must report, the people who must report to you, those whom you supervise, and those with whom you work directly, all have formal communication relationships that will show up on an accurate organizational chart. (See Figure 5.1 for an example of an organizational chart.)

The three major forms of formal message flow are *downward communication, upward communication*, and *horizontal communication*. All three of these forms of message flow follow the relationships between organization members prescribed by the organizational chart, and all three forms of message flow perform important functions for the organization.

Downward communication flows from upper management down to lower levels in the organizational hierarchy. Downward communication is the most basic type of formal message system. Several of the key organizational

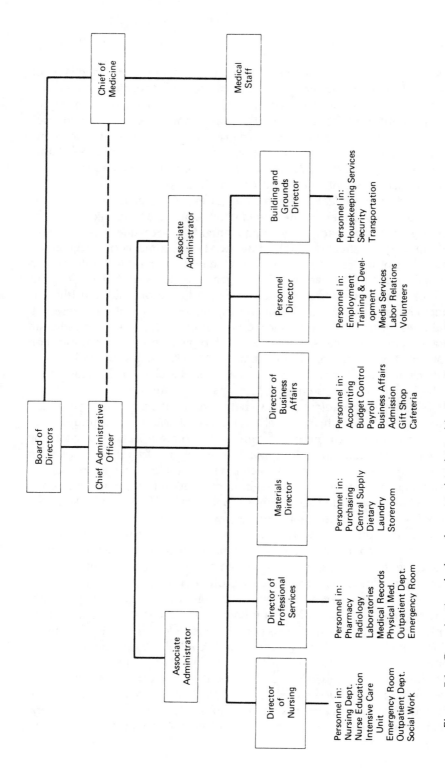

Figure 5.1 Organizational chart for a Mythical Health Care Organization

functions of downward communication include sending orders, giving job related information, reviewing job performance, and indoctrinating members toward organizational goals. Downward communication is an important management tool for directing the performance of workers in their organizational tasks. There is usually a great abundance of downward communication in health care organizations. As we will discuss in more depth, however, the prevalence of downward communication messages does not imply *effective* use of downward communication.

Upward communication flows from lower level employees within the organization up to management personnel. Upward communication is the primary source of feedback to management. The feedback is useful for determining the effectiveness of downward communication. Additionally, upward communication messages provide management with information about the day-to-day operation of the organization to use in making decisions and for encouraging employee participation in the organization (thereby enhancing organizational cohesiveness and relieving employee tensions). Channels for upward communication are often underdeveloped in health care organizations causing a variety of organizational communication problems for the delivery of health care. We will discuss the problems of insufficient upward communication later on in this chapter. The case study at the beginning of this chapter provides one example.

Horizontal communication flows between members of the organization who are at the same hierarchical level; it is basically peer communication between organization members. Horizontal communication functions by allowing task coordination, providing a means for sharing relevant information, as well as providing a channel for problem solving and conflict maintenance. Although horizontal communication is an important formal channel of organizational communication it is often overlooked and underused in organizational practice.

Even though downward, upward, and horizontal channels of organizational communication provide important communication functions, in practice, formal message flow is often poorly utilized. Downward communication, although heavily utilized, is often overplayed by management. In chapter 2 we differentiated between content and relationship aspects of messages. In downward communication the content information of explaining procedures and goals can be overshadowed by the relationship information of establishing power and control. Overdependence on continually giving orders and instructions to workers can alienate workers from management, causing employee resentment toward management and the organization. Downward communication is often unclear and contradictory, causing confusion and anxiety for organization members. Later in this chapter we will discuss the problems of contradictory downward communication messages in health care organizations, which causes role conflict for many health care workers.

There are several factors in organizations that cause upward communication channels to be underdeveloped. Since people higher up in the organizational hierarchy wield power over those people holding lower positions within the organizations, it is very risky for workers to tell their bosses about problems that exist in the organization or about gripes they have with management's downward communication. If a worker's upward communication evokes the wrath of his or her boss, the worker's job might be jeopardized. Because of the risks involved with the upward disclosure of unpopular information, workers often communicate only favorable messages to their bosses, a syndrome known as the *mum effect*. Moreover, management is often unreceptive to honest employee feedback and reacts angrily and defensively to upward communication. The story about the ancient Greek monarch who would slay the messengers who brought him unfavorable news about military campaigns is similar to the more current story about a nurse who informed hospital management about questionable health care procedures leading to a baby's death and was fired for her troubles. Such situations strongly discourage other hospital workers from coming to management with unfavorable information.

The greatest problem with horizontal communication in most organizations is management's failure to recognize it as being useful. In many organizations, peer communication is discouraged and sometimes results in punishment. Horizontal communication is often thought of as merely being small talk and fraternizing between workers. At management levels, organization members often become so busy working within their own area of the organization they have little time for communicating with other personnel at their same hierarchical level. Yet, as we discussed earlier, horizontal communication provides organization members with useful information allowing them to solve problems and coordinate activities.

To utilize downward, upward, and horizontal message flow in organizations effectively, management must become aware of the importance of formal message flow in their organization. Downward messages must be clear, informative, and sensitive to prepare organization members for organizational tasks without being patronizing. Management must demonstrate genuine receptiveness to open and honest upward communication in order to obtain the vital feedback necessary to direct organizational performance. Workers should be encouraged to share their ideas with management. After all, those health care workers directly involved with the performance of organizational tasks know firsthand what works and what doesn't work in health care practice. Management can tap into the knowledge of health care workers by eliciting feedback. Horizontal communication between organization members should be encouraged by management especially in complex situations where task coordination and problem-solving skills are most necessary.

Some communication strategies for improving formal message flow in organizations include the use of group meetings to facilitate interaction among organization members, regular performance review and problem-solving interviews between management and workers, formal training procedures and orientation programs for workers, suggestion boxes and worker idea reward systems, as well as briefing sessions during shift changes. Organizational media such as newsletters, memos, taped messages, training films, and bulletin boards can be used to augment formal message flow in organizations. However, the key to effective formal message flow in organizations, whether it be downward, upward, or horizontal, is the development of meaningful interpersonal relationships between organization members. Only through the development of effective human relationships can organization members learn how to trust one another and to communicate meaningfully with each other.

In addition to formal message flow systems that have been prescribed by the formal hierarchy of the organization, an informal message flow system emerges naturally through human interaction within the organization. *Informal message flow* refers to the communication that develops between organization members that is not necessarily prescribed by the formal goals and hierarchy of the organization but develops out of interpersonal attraction, shared social interests, and nontask-oriented interaction among organization members. As we mentioned, informal message flow does not necessarily follow the organizational hierarchy but instead develops its own social structure. Often this informal channel of communication in organizations is referred to as the *grapevine* and is usually composed of social groups, cliques, club members, family relations, and other informal relationships that develop between organization members.

One of the primary reasons for the development of informal communication systems within organizations is the need organization members have for information about the organization. Organizations are often large, complex, and multifaceted systems. In order for members of organizations to behave effectively within their organizations, they need information about what is going on behind the scenes and what is being planned by other members. The grapevine provides organization members with information about who is doing what and what changes are occurring within the organization, affording information about organizational functioning that can help them direct their activities.

In organizations information is powerful. Whoever possesses information about the organization and is willing to barter that information can exercise power within that organization. Often individuals who seek organizational power, especially those who are not afforded power through the formal organizational hierarchy, attempt to gain power by gathering information through their activities within the grapevine. Those organization members who possess a great deal of information and utilize their information to direct the grapevine are known as *informal leaders.*

Informal leaders wield a great deal of power within organizations, yet, strangely enough, they are seldom recognized by the formal power structure of the organization as being either legitimate or powerful. Due to this management oversight, the formal and informal systems within the organization are often in competition with one another. For years organizational theorists have been planning to stamp out the grapevine, not realizing the grapevine is a naturally developing part of organizations based on human beings' quest for organizational information. Paradoxically, the more strongly the management attempts to rid itself of the grapevine, the more it grows and flourishes. This was exemplified by the case study at the beginning of the chapter. The more uncertain and turbulent the communication climate of the organization becomes, the more organization members feel the need for information about the organization.

A more effective strategy for utilizing the informal message flow in organizations is to coordinate formal and informal communication systems. Organization members usually become informal leaders because of their extreme desire for power and recognition within the organization, often known as *Machiavellian* tendencies. Management can feed the Machiavellian tendencies of their organization's informal leaders by keeping these leaders informed about important happenings in the organization and by developing a trusting relationship with them. By feeding these informal leaders with honest and important information about the organization, management can enlist these leaders and their informal channels of communication to spread information through the organization, supplementing formal downward message flow channels. Furthermore, management can elicit useful upward communication from the informal leaders, who know a great deal about organizational operations. Perhaps even more importantly, management can eliminate the spread of dangerously untrue rumors and replace them with organizationally approved information on the grapevine.

In the case history at the beginning of this chapter, Horace Jackson was identified as an informal leader in the hospital. Although his formal position was that of a janitor, his informal position was extremely influential due to the information he had gathered and relationships he had developed working at the hospital for more than thirty years. When the new hospital administrator ignored Horace, he was really ignoring the informal communication system within the hospital. Since the new administrator wasn't cultivating the grapevine and feeding it with accurate information, Horace took it upon himself to feed the grapevine with false information, information about massive layoffs at the hospital. Eventually the new administrator was made aware of the importance of the informal communication system in the hospital and began to integrate formal and informal organizational communication systems by providing Horace with relevant and accurate organizational information.

Role Conflict and Multiple Authority in Health Care

Hospitals have developed as the primary health care organizations in the modern world. As such, they embody the wide variety of health care personnel, technologies, and services that are part of the modern health care system. In the delivery of health care services, the activities of many individuals are coordinated, necessitating the development of extensive administrative and control systems in hospital organizations. In fact, many hospitals tend to become top-heavy. That is, hospital organizations often develop disproportionately extensive hierarchies of control. The overdevelopment of hierarchical levels in health care organizations contributes to the development of several administrative problems for health care workers.

As House (1970) points out, the overdevelopment of hospital hierarchies violates two basic principles of management, *chain of command* and *unity of command*. The principle of chain of command asserts that organizations should have a clear hierarchy of control where each level of the organization holds the responsibility for directing the activities of people at lower levels, with authority flowing directly from the top of the organization to the bottom. The principle of unity of command relates closely to chain of command, asserting that within organizational hierarchies subordinates should receive a command from only one supervisor to minimize confusion in directing organizational activities.

In hospital organizations there are usually at least two major sources of control — hospital administration and medical administration. Additionally, the professional standards of each of the health practitioners, whether they be pharmacists, physicians, nurses, dentists, therapists, or social workers, in effect, directs the performance of health care professionals. These different sources of hierarchical control complicate the direction of organizational activities. The hospital chain of command is often bypassed because of the many sources of control. For example, a physician who is not a full-time member of the hospital staff but is there treating one of his or her clients may order a nurse to treat that client in a manner that is contradictory to the general rules of hospital administration or medical administration. The nurse is put into a double bind and must decide whether to disregard the doctor's instructions and perhaps jeopardize the well-being of the client or follow the doctor's orders and violate the regulations of the hospital administration. The nurse may wonder who is in control in that situation. Must he or she answer to the doctor, to the hospital administration, or to personal professional judgment? The chain of command is not clear and can cause ambiguity and frustration that may result in health care activities that do not meet the standards of all parties concerned.

In the same health care situation, unity of command may also be violated. The nurse is given mutually contradictory orders by the medical staff, the administrative staff, and perhaps the nursing hierarchy as well. This puts the nurse in a classic double bind situation. No matter what the nurse decides to do, at least one of his or her bosses' instructions will be disobeyed.

The situation of multiple authority in health care organizations puts many health care workers in an untenable situation where they are uncertain about their health care duties and their health care roles. This uncertainty about the clear definition of the health practitioner's role is known as *role ambiguity*. Role ambiguity results from unclear and ambiguous information about how the professional is to do his or her job. *Role congruence* is the degree to which the health practitioner's job performance matches the role expectations of both administrator and practitioner. Certainly in situations of multiple authority the health care organization suffers from insufficient role congruence. Lack of role congruence, in turn, puts the health practitioner in a situation of *role conflict*, where the practitioner is caught between two or more mutually exclusive expectations for job performance. Of course, all organizational members have a certain amount of role conflict in the performance of their jobs, due to differing expectations. In health care organizations, role conflict abounds. Employee frustration, confusion, and, in many cases, poor job performance are the results.

The problem of multiple authority and role conflict in health care organizations is a clear situation of too many chefs and too few cooks. There are too many people giving orders about the administration of health care to a small number of health care workers. This situation is caused by the growing complexity of the health care delivery system. As health care knowledge develops, new specialized areas of health care practice are added to the repertoire of hospital services, increasing the number of specialized personnel and administrators to coordinate their activities in the health care organization. The ever-increasing specialization of health care practice has resulted in the growing departmentalization and decentralization of health care delivery organizations. Health care organizations generally have many middle management personnel wielding a rather narrow *span of control* over the limited number of health care personnel they directly supervise. Narrow span of control is a characteristic of *decentralization*, while *centralized organizations* usually have fewer bosses sharing the responsibility of directing the activities of many subordinates. Generally, a centralized organization has a narrow chain of command, while a decentralized organization has many different divisions, each with management personnel who have formal organizational responsibility. Centralized organizations have relatively few power and decision points, while decentralized organizations have many points where formal power is wielded and decisions are made.

Decentralization is often advantageous for complex organizations because it relieves the extreme organizational responsibilities of top management, spreading decision-making responsibility among middle managers who are directly involved in the operation of the organization. Certainly decentralization is beneficial in health care organizations such as hospitals because it puts the responsibility for specialized health care decision making on the health care professionals who are most knowledgeable about and more involved with the specific health care situation.

On the other side, however, decentralization has the disadvantage of giving middle managers decision-making responsibilities when they often do not see the larger organizational picture and the implications of their decisions on other organizational divisions or personnel. In health care organizations, the decision makers are often so involved with their own immediate health care delivery problems they may not recognize the repercussions of their decisions on the rest of the hospital. Moreover, as we have already pointed out, since health care areas overlap in the delivery of health care services, there is great opportunity for contradictory decisions and directives from different sources of authority in decentralized health care organizations. Once again, multiple authority in health care can lead to role conflict, which in turn can lead to frustration, confusion, and inefficient health care services.

Decentralization, multiple authority, and role conflict have become an inevitable part of organizational life in health care practice. To minimize the problems of role conflict in organizations, several authors have suggested the use of management personnel to serve as integrators and liaisons in complex organizations (Cassella, 1977; Fisher, 1981; Kreps, 1990a). These integrators will help connect the different divisions of the organization, allowing specialists to understand the larger picture implications of their specialized decisions. Ombudspeople, or people appointed to hear, investigate and ameliorate complaints of organization members, can often help health care personnel work out role conflicts between them and their supervisors. Communication between health care personnel across hospital divisions and hierarchical levels can break down role conflict and help foster cooperation between members of the health care organizations.

Coping with Organizational Bureaucracy

The ever increasing complexity and specialization of health care delivery has caused health care organizations to become very bureaucratic. *Bureaucracy* refers to the level of formalization of rules and processes within an organization. Although in modern word usage bureaucracy has gotten a bad name, classical organizational theorists have for many years advocated bureaucratic models for administering organizations (Fayol, 1949). The bureaucratic organization exhibits the following characteristics: *rules* and regulations, *division of labor, hierarchy* of formal organizational power, *interchangeability of personnel in relatively self-perpetuating organizational roles, impersonality* in interpersonal relationships, and *rationality* and predictability in the accomplishment of organizational goals. Modern health care organizations are designed to embody these characteristics of bureaucracy.

The bureaucratic model has gotten a bad public image in recent years due to extreme formality of bureaucratic organizations. The word bureaucracy has become almost synonymous with organizational inefficiency, red tape and insensitivity. Bradley and Baird (1980) report that "complaints against bureaucracy have been numerous: it has been accused of stifling individual creativity, encouraging conformity and modifying the personality," (p.10). Certainly hospitals have had many of these same criticisms leveled at them. Health care organizations are notorious for their red tape. Stories of dying patients who were denied treatment in public hospitals until they filled out forms or identified their method of payment or insurance abound. Stories like these attest not only to the red tape and insensitivity of bureaucracies but also to the ways that the overdevelopment of bureaucratic structures can become self-defeating to the accomplishment of organizational goals.

Bureaucracy, however, offers many advantages to large complex organizations such as hospitals. Precision, speed, clarity, continuity, discretion, unity, and strict subordination of personnel are reported as benefits of bureaucratic structure (Kreps, 1990a). Bureaucratic structure adds predictability to organizational behavior by prescribing rules and procedures for dealing with tasks. Rules help organizations cope with routine problems. Bureaucracy is useful for handling normal, predictable organizational tasks. Yet, rules are not useful in responding to very complex situations, suggesting the bureaucratic model is inappropriate for use in response to complex organizational problems. Bureaucracy does not lend itself to creativity, yet many hospitals must react creatively to the unpredictable health care problems presented to them by consumers. In retrospect, bureaucracy can offer many strong advantages to organizational practice, yet can also be very constraining for the organization.

The strengths and limitations of bureaucracy for organizational functioning underscore the ongoing tension in organizations between *differentiation* and *integration*. Differentiation refers to the needs organizations have for specialized personnel and processes. Health care organizations utilize specialized health professionals, technologies, and procedures in the delivery of health care services, thereby exhibiting differentiation. Integration refers to the needs organizations have for coordinating the many different activities and processes of organizing in achieving their goals. Hospitals strive to coordinate the activities of doctors, nurses, pharmacists, therapists, support staff, and clients in the delivery of health care services, thereby exhibiting integration. Differentiation and integration are often mutually competing processes in organizations. The more differentiated (specialized and departmentalized) a health care organization is, the more difficult it becomes for the organization to demonstrate integration (coordination and cooperation). Conversely, the more integrated an organization is, the more difficult it is for the organization to differentiate. In a similar manner bureaucracy helps an organization respond in regulated, ordered, predictable ways but often makes it difficult for organizations to develop innovative patterns and processes.

Organizations must develop a workable balance between differentiation and integration to remain viable, and they also must maintain a healthy balance between bureaucracy (structure) and adaptability (flexibility and creativity). The organizational balance between differentiation and integration and between bureaucracy and adaptability is achieved through the ongoing maintenance, evaluation, and development of organizational processes by management. The formal organization leaders should continually seek feedback from organization members, as well as from customers (in health care the management should seek feedback from clients) to evaluate the function and relational effectiveness of organizational processes and structures, utilizing the information gathered to update and develop the organization so it may operate more effectively in the future.

On an individual level, organization members can best cope with the rigidity and impersonality of highly formalized health care bureaucracies by becoming familiar with the rules and regulations and hierarchical power relationships that make up the bureaucratic structure of the system. By learning the "ropes" of the system, individuals can utilize organizational structure to their best advantage. Knowing who has the authority and power to get things done in an organization, as well as finding out the procedures and mechanisms for initiating changes and facilitating organizational action can help the organization member achieve personal, professional, and task related goals within the organization. As we mentioned earlier in this chapter, information is extremely powerful in organizations; knowing with whom to speak and what channels to utilize in an organization can be very powerful information for an individual to possess. Additionally, the development of good working relationships with fellow organization members at all levels of the hierarchy can help an individual achieve his or her goals. It is especially useful to establish communication relationships with formal and informal organization leaders who can provide other members with important information about the operation, the present condition and future actions of the organization. By learning the rules and structures of the organization and establishing effective interpersonal relationships with organization members, individuals can help direct activities within bureaucratic organizations, rather than be manipulated by the bureaucracy.

Bureaucratic regulations provide relevant information for directing health care activities and help maintain order within the health care organization on a content level. On a relationship level, however, the proliferation of rules and regulations in health care organizations can be stifling and dehumanizing, especially for health care consumers who often pay dearly in both time and money to seek health care services. For many health care consumers, hospitalization is tantamount to incarceration (Kreps, 1990b; Mendelsohn, 1979). The many rules in health care organizations that govern patient behavior limit the social potential of the individual and tend to reinforce the *sick role*. Health care consumers often feel stifled and frustrated.

Institutionalization often has a dehumanizing influence on health care clients, especially long-term care patients such as elderly residents of nursing homes (Mendelson, 1974; Kreps, 1990b). Entry into health care systems, such as hospitals or nursing homes, severely constrain elders' freedom of choice. As a client, the elder is generally "assigned" a patient number, a patient chart, a bed, a room, a medical regimen, and sometimes even given institutionally approved garments to wear. Elders must adapt to the health care system's schedule of events rather than be able to choose their own schedule of activities, including when to eat, when to sleep, and when to use the toilet. Daily events are often scheduled for the client, with little or no heed for the individual's wishes. For example, elderly nursing home residents are often given little choice about what foods they want to eat; dieticians make those choices for them. Hospital personnel take the elder for lab tests, therapy sessions, and even surgical operations according to a schedule prepared for the client, often with little or no collaboration with the elder. The elder is regularly told when to sit up, when to lie down, when to stand up. Strong evidence indicates the institutionalization of health care delivery in many organizations can limit the effectiveness of health care treatment by alienating and dehumanizing health care recipients (U.S. Senate Special Committee on Aging, Subcommittee on Long Term Care, 1974; 1975).

Just as health care employees can cope with organizational bureaucracy by becoming more familiar with the norms and rules of the health care system, clients can also attempt to overcome the red tape and inefficiency of health care bureaucracies by becoming informed consumers who are aware of their rights as clients and who are actively involved in directing their own health care. Often, if consumers are not well-informed about the intricate workings of health care systems, it is useful for the client to enlist the help of knowledgeable family members, friends, or health care providers to serve as their *advocates* within the health care system. Advocates can help seek relevant information for consumers from health care administrators and providers, solve administrative snafus and problems, and make sure that the client's wishes are heard when treatment decisions are made. Clients (working individually or with the help of advocates) who are aware of hospital rules, regulations, and procedures are in a good position to direct their own health care because they understand the workings of the health care system which helps them to act strategically. Knowledge about the health care system also helps to minimize the intimidation, confusion, and dehumanization consumers often experience when dealing with complex and unwieldy hospital bureaucracies.

Health Care Organizations as Information Processors

Organizations are social structures that facilitate adaptation by helping people interpret and respond appropriately to the many challenging and complex information situations that confront them (Kreps, 1990a; Weick, 1979). Health care organizations help members and clients adapt to environmental constraints and cope with complex problems they encounter. For example, health care organizations provide consumers with information processing resources to help them understand and solve their health problems. In a very real sense, coping with threats to individual health is an information processing problem for most people since serious health problems are often too equivocal (complex, confusing, and unpredictable) for individuals to fully interpret, understand, and adequately respond to by themselves (Zola, 1963). Health care providers seek relevant information through their organizational affiliations to help them understand the many health problems facing clients, to navigate through a complex and bureaucratic health care system, and to coordinate interdependent health care activities.

Health care consumers need specialized information to direct their health preserving activities. With the help of knowledgeable others, provided from within the health care organization, consumers can cope with complex health threats. The more equivocal health problems are, the more equivocal health care processes for interpreting and effectively responding to these problems must be (the *principle of requisite variety*), and the more likely consumers are to need the information processing resources of health care organizations (Weick, 1979). Routine health care ailments, such as headaches or common colds, pose less complex information processing problems, necessitating less information processing power than an acute, highly equivocal health care problem like a brain tumor. Equivocal problems demand the information processing resources of a health care organization — tests have to be conducted; specialists must be consulted; complex treatments and operations may have to be performed. Only health care organizations, with well-trained personnel and specialized equipment, can help clients cope with highly equivocal health care problems.

Members of health care organizations also need specialized information to perform their jobs effectively. In the case at the beginning of this chapter, Horace had performed an important information processing job for members of the hospital — that is, until the new administrator came on board. Prior to the arrival of the new administrator, Horace had provided other employees with relevant inside information about the organization and its membership. This information helped the employees understand what was going on within the organization and decide how they could respond to new organizational situations. Of course, in this case, Horace deliberately passed on erroneous information to discredit the new hospital administrator. The fact, however, that most people believed the rumor Horace spread demonstrates his power as a trusted source of information within the organization. This trust will not last long if he continues to misinform other members of the organization. Horace is a powerful contact within the hospital because he is normally a very good source of inside information. The negative rumor not only threatened the new administrator but also threatened Horace's informal position within the organization.

The following case, "The Hospital as an Information System," further illustrates the information needs of modern health care organizations. Hospitals are excellent examples of organizations that are exceptionally dependent on timely and accurate information. Any slight information delay or distortion can have life-threatening repercussions for health care consumers. The case describes a potentially dangerous organizational situation where the hospital information system breaks down, causing a serious dilemma for hospital employees and patients. As you read the general background and the specifics of this case, try to identify the different sources of information on which the hospital must rely. How well are these information sources being utilized in this organization? How can the information needed by organization members be effectively gathered, interpreted, stored, and provided in the hospital? How might this health care organization's information system be improved?

The Hospital as an Information System*

A perceptive visitor to a hospital would observe that a great deal of staff activity is devoted to information processing activities.

Several nurses are at the nursing station filling out patient record forms, talking on the telephone, or discussing the coordination of their day's schedule. A doctor is being paged on a P.A. system. Food trays are being wheeled down the corridor to patients' rooms. Each tray was assigned to a specific patient on the basis of particular dietary needs, as indicated on a form that was sent previously to the hospital kitchen. At bedside, a doctor is obtaining information from a patient about symptoms. This information will then be entered in the patient's record file.

It would be hard to overestimate the importance of this file to the hospital. If the record file were ever lost or misplaced, as sometimes happens, the hospital would be at almost a complete loss as to how to treat the patient. The file originates when the patient enters the hospital's door, and it must accompany the patient wherever he or she goes: to x-ray or to surgery, for example. Upon discharge, the file (by this time an inch or two thick with forms, charts, and notes, which represent hundreds of hours of skilled expertise worth thousands of dollars) is placed in the hospital records department where it will remain permanently. The record file is so sacred to the hospital that the patient is not allowed to see it, except in very unusual cases, and then only with the permission of the doctor. The file can be so thick that it becomes an information overload problem. One solution is to computerize the file data; another approach is to utilize a "problem-oriented" record system in which essential data are isolated and instantly accessible.

Great effort is expended by the hospital to ensure that the patient record file contains adequate and accurate information. Each entry in the file must be signed and initialed so that responsibility for it is precisely fixed. Every bit of information about the patient must be recorded: every bowel movement, every medication that is administered, every rise in temperature. The cost of an error in the patient file is catastrophic. Each year one or more patients' deaths in a typical hospital may be caused by errors in information processing or transmittal. To prevent such monumental errors most hospitals expend great effort on continually redesigning their communication systems, on training and retraining the hospital staff to use them properly, and on checking accuracy and adequacy through various feedback devices.

Despite such extensive precautions, however, embarrassing communication breakdowns still occur. One spectacular sample is the case of a patient in the Chicago-area Veterans Administration hospital, Erwin Pawelski, who was "lost" for twenty-seven hours.

Pawelski, a paralyzed patient who could not speak, was strapped onto a wheelchair by an attendant and wheeled out of his ward to receive occupational therapy at 9:30 A.M. on May 1, 1975. What happened next is anybody's guess. The patient record file shows a twenty-seven hour blank. A hospital spokesman later told newspaper reporters: "There's a presumption that he arrived in the basement for therapy. But we are not positive."

At 7:00 A.M. on May 2nd, Pawelski's wife was called by the hospital to ask if she had removed him from the hospital. When she rushed to the hospital, she found that another patient had moved into his bed. Pawelski's effects had been shoved into a closet.

Pawelski was found by a therapy supervisor who stepped into an elevator in the hospital basement at 1:10 P.M. on May 2nd. The hospital has 3,000 employees, 1,295 patients, and about 700 visitors daily. Pawelski was in one of the main banks of elevators, ridden each day by hundreds of doctors, nurses, attendants, patients, and visitors. "It's unbelievable that there wouldn't be one person during those twenty-seven hours offering to help this man slumped over in a wheelchair. It's a mystery what happened," stated the hospital spokesman.

Twenty days after Pawelski was "misplaced" for twenty-seven hours, he died from cerebral hemorrhage after undergoing brain surgery. The hospital claimed the death was not connected with any ill effects sustained from the incident.

A hospital can best be viewed, then, as an organization that devotes much of its activity to processing information. So, in fact, do most other types of organizations.

This case clearly illustrates the importance of gathering, interpreting, preserving, and making available relevant information in health care organizations. Information is the resource that is used to direct health care activities, and human communication is the process by which relevant health information is generated and shared. Effective human communication is crucially important in organizing activities. As health knowledge has increased, health care services have become more complex. There is a pronounced need for organizations to help handle the management of health information. Effective communication of relevant information, often with the use of computerized communication systems, aids organizations in adapting to ever-changing health care issues. Adaptation of health care organizations to emergent health information constraints facilitates viable health care service delivery in the modern world.

Optimally, health care organizations should provide the communication structure, personnel, and technology for coping with complex health care situations. There were some obvious communication problems in the VA hospital depicted in this case history. Try to identify and analyze the specific communication-related issues which caused problems in this situation. Based upon the information you were provided in this case, see if you can answer the following questions:

1. What is meant when this hospital is characterized as being an information system? Identify the key elements of this hospital information system.

2. What are the communication functions of this hospital information system? Are these information functions typical of health care organizations?

3. Identify some of the primary sources of information in this hospital. How is the information gathered from these sources and later processed and stored in the hospital information system? How can the information be retrieved by hospital members?

4. What role does communication play in the hospital information system? How has this relationship between communication and information led to organizational problems in the case?

5. Identify some of the communication problems evident in this hospital. What could be done to improve the communication/information system in this organization? Optimally, how should this system work?

6. Do you believe the hospital spokesperson's claim that the information breakdown experienced in this case had no relation to Pawelski's demise? How do you think this experience may have affected Pawelski? What implications does this suggest about the importance of accurate and timely information in health care organizations?

7. What role could a patient advocate have performed for Mr. Pawelski in this case?

Internal and External Organizational Communication

Information flow in health care organizations must be directed and coordinated internally and eternally for organizations to function effectively (Kreps, 1990a). Health care organizations are complex social systems composed of networks of interdependent groups of health care providers, support staff, and consumers — all the activities of these groups must be coordinated (Perrow, 1965). Health care administrators direct internal organizational information flow between different departments and divisions to coordinate health preserving and administrative activities of the system (Pfeffer & Salancik, 1977).

How well did the new administrator in the case at the beginning of this chapter direct the internal information flow in his hospital? He was oblivious to the fact that the informal information system in the hospital was contradicting everything he was communicating through the formal communication system. In solving this problem, the consultant helped the new administrator coordinate formal and informal channels of internal communication. How well did the administrators in the VA hospital in the "Hospital as an Information System" case direct internal information flow? What could they have done to avoid the problems they encountered by "misplacing" Mr. Pawelski? Do you think that implementation of a patient monitoring communication system (where each department would keep records about when and where clients entered, left, and were scheduled to arrive at the department, as well as who had the responsibility for transporting clients) would help reduce the chances that such problems might occur or, at the very least, increase the hospital's ability to locate clients?

Interprofessional relationships between the many different providers in health care organizations must be managed. Ineffective interprofessional relationships between health care providers is a major problem in health care delivery systems (Hill, 1978; Kindig, 1975; Frank, 1961; Boyer, Lee, & Kirschner, 1977). Power and status discrepancies between practitioners can lead to professional domination and conflict between health care providers (Friedson, 1970). Differences in education, orientation to health care, and evaluations of other health care disciplines can make interprofessional relations uneasy. In Chapter 7, Culture and Health Communication, we will examine how different health care professional groups socialize their members into professional cultures. These cultural influences often cause health care professionals to be ethnocentric about the legitimacy of their profession in comparison to other health care professional groups. Conflict often occurs over domain consensus and authority due to the overlapping responsibilities and interdependent activities of the various health care providers (Starr, 1982).

Not only do health care professionals have professional cultures, but every health care organization also has its own unique cultural identity. The history of the organization and the unique combination of individuals which comprise it help shape an organization's identity. The primary ingredient of *organizational culture* is the collective interpretations organization members make about organizational activities and the outcomes of these activities. Examples would be the meanings that hospital employees assign to hospital products, technologies and tools; interpretations about identities and character traits of well-known physicians or administrators; the significance of uniforms and dress codes for different personnel in the hospital; designation of hospital property, buildings, and architectural design; as well as interpretations about the legitimacy of organizational rules that govern formal activities. The interpretive frameworks provided in organizational cultures combine to form unique *cultural themes* that direct organization members' actions. These themes influence member attitudes and values, the specialized jargons and languages they use, social and professional rituals they engage in, company history and philosophies that are passed on, legends, stories and jokes that are told, informal norms and logics used to guide actions, visions organization members have of the organization's future, and the identification of organizational friends and foes.

The stronger a cultural theme is, the larger the percentage of organization members who abide by it. Strong cultural themes can be either productive or destructive since these themes have powerful influences on both the interpretations organization members make about reality and the activities in which they engage. *Productive cultural themes* can help promote organizational growth and development. For example, at the National Cancer Institute, there is a strong productive cultural belief that the institute's programs are saving thousands of lives by "winning the war on cancer." Scientists often devote all of their available time and energy to conduct their research programs. (Institute scientists routinely work days and evenings, over weekends, and through vacation periods to achieve their research goals.) *Destructive cultural themes* can work to the detriment of the organization. For example, in the case at the beginning of the chapter the rumor that Horace spread about the new administrator became a strong negative cultural theme that led to problems with staff morale and probably decreased the quality of health care services within the organization.

Human communication is the primary channel used to promote the development and maintenance of organizational culture. There is a very close relationship between organizational communication and organizational culture since communication provides organization members with information and socializes members into the organization's culture (Pacanowsky and O'Donnell-Trujillo, 1982; Kreps, 1990a). Organizational culture is communicated to health care employees and relevant others informally through interpersonal storytelling and gossiping using the organization's grapevine as a primary medium. Culture is communicated formally through the use of hospital advertising, slogans, documents (such as newsletters, annual reports, handbooks, and other company publications), group meetings, and public presentations.

As an organization's identity emerges, members interpret the organization's past and present, making sense of the phenomena of organizational life and creating stories and legends about organizational activities. These stories and legends provide a thematic base for the organization. Culturally derived explanations about what the organization is, development of collective visions about the future development of what it will do, how it goes about accomplishing its goals, and what role organization members play in these activities comprise organizational folklore and are essential elements in the development of an organizational identity (Kreps, 1990a).

Stories and inside jokes are often used by organization members to illustrate cultural themes. For example, at a large county hospital whose name had been changed from "County General" to "Wishard Memorial," there was a cultural theme held by hospital employees that the general public had not kept up with advancements and improvements made at the hospital and held an unrealistically poor image of the hospital. A joke was told among the hospital staff that illustrated this theme. The joke tells about an emergency patient brought to the hospital while unconscious. When the client woke up, he worriedly asked a nurse, "Where am I?" The nurse replied, "You are at Wishard Memorial Hospital." The client gave a sigh of relief and responded, "Thank goodness I'm not at County General." To fully appreciate this joke you have to understand the theme about the unwarranted negative public image of the hospital. This story reinforces the accepted cultural theme about an uninformed public, while demonstrating to hospital employees how unrealistic the negative public image is.

The potential benefits of organizational culture in helping organization members both interpret and respond appropriately to complex organizational phenomena can be of great utility to modern organizations. When knowledge of the benefits of productive cultural themes is coupled with recognition of the role of organizational communication as a pervasive channel for socialization several directions for enlightened organizational practice become apparent. Health care organization administrators can utilize formal and informal communication channels to educate their members about their organizational culture, to socialize them into the culture, and eventually to develop a strong organizational culture.

Formal organizational communication channels such as advertising, slogans, annual reports, newsletters, written correspondence, internal company documents, group meetings, and speeches should be designed to promote the development of organizational culture. Cultural values, company history, organizational heroes, significant cultural symbols, and cultural visions for the organization's future can be presented to the organization's relevant publics through formal communication. Orientation programs as well as in-house training and development programs can be designed to help health care employees learn about their organization's culture. These information programs will help employees identify more fully with both the organization and their co-workers and will help them direct their organizational activities in accordance with cultural norms.

Informal communication can also be used to promote organizational culture, although the grapevine can be more difficult to direct than formal communication channels. As we discussed earlier in this chapter, management often concentrates solely on formal communication channels, either avoiding the informal communication or allowing it to develop on its own. Informal communication channels, however, can be integrated with formal communication channels in organizations, developing a complementary overlap between the formal and informal information carried throughout the organization. Health care administrators can help direct the grapevine by providing its informal leaders with culturally relevant information.

Strong cultures can facilitate increased member solidarity and cohesiveness by enabling cultural constituents to identify with each other and with their organization. Increased member identification and knowledge often lead to improved cooperation and coordination among organization members, something that is essential for effective health care systems. Awareness of cultural information can also help organization members develop enhanced abilities to utilize *organizational intelligence* (information about how to get things done in an organization) in guiding their organizational activities. In the "Hospital as an Information System" case, it appears that the culture of the organization did not promote high levels of cooperation, coordination, nor organizational intelligence among hospital staff. Perhaps the hospital had a negative cultural theme that encouraged hospital employees to be concerned only with their own clients and activities and not to get involved with other departments' business. In a more cooperative organizational culture, when Mr. Pawelski did not arrive at the occupational therapy department as scheduled, a department representative would have called Mr. Pawelski's ward to find out where he was. At a minimum, a representative from the ward would have called the occupational therapy department when Mr. Pawelski did not arrive back at the ward. In a strong cooperative organizational culture, any one of the hundreds of employees that must have passed Mr. Pawelski while he was in the elevator would have felt the personal responsibility to find out why this paralyzed man was there. Even though he was not their client, they would have made sure he was returned to his room. Health care administrators must be aware of the cultural beliefs and values that exist within their organization and use communication strategies to promote productive cultural themes and minimize negative cultural themes.

In addition to directing internal communications, managing interprofessional relations, and developing productive organizational cultures, health care system administrators must also be able to go beyond the boundaries of their organizations to provide relevant information to key publics and to gather information for making strategic decisions to guide their health care organizations. For example, fund raising, lobbying, personnel recruitment, and media relations are all potentially important functions of external information systems in health care organizations (Pfeffer, 1973; Kreps, 1990a). Effective health care administrators proactively direct their organizations' interaction with its relevant environment. *Proactive* management means planning ahead to avoid or cope with problems before the problems damage the organization. A proactive health care system administrator will routinely gather relevant information from the health care organization's relevant environment about imminent health care problems and plan organizational strategies for meeting these potential problems. For example, the development of specialized triage methods for processing and treating flood victims in an area where there are flood plains and flooding is a strong possibility for the future. It might be too late to develop and implement these specialized procedures at the time of a major flood. Having these procedures available helps prepare the health care organization to cope effectively with the health care demands of its environment. How proactive were the administrators in the two cases in this chapter? What could they have done to become more proactive?

Organizations, like human beings, must be able to adapt to survive. Administrators of health care organizations constantly need feedback from internal and external information sources about the performance of their organizations to identify performance gaps and initiate constructive change (Rogers & Agarwala-Rogers, 1976). A *performance gap* is the difference between what an organization intends to accomplish and what it actually does accomplish. Since all organizations experience performance gaps, it is important to identify and monitor those gaps to help the organization work toward achieving unfulfilled goals.

Important sources of feedback for an organization are its members, especially those who work with consumers (cosmopolites) since they can provide the organization with information about both the internal environment, to which they belong, and the external environment, with which they have daily contact. In the case at the beginning of the chapter, the consultant was able to diagnose the causes of low morale in the hospital by seeking information (feedback) from hospital employees. He learned about the rumors being spread through the hospital and was able to identify the source of the rumors by interacting with the people who were most knowledgeable about the organization — its members. These communication contacts provided the consultant with valuable information about the current state of the organization.

Leaders of many health care organizations, just as in the case at the beginning of this chapter, often fail to recognize and fully utilize the information resources their employees possess (Kreps, 1990a). Can you imagine how much relevant information about hospital activities the new administrator in this case could have acquired from Horace by establishing an effective communication relationship with this informal leader? He might have avoided the entire morale problem that developed in the hospital by exchanging relevant information with Horace. Administrative neglect of the information needs of and information resources available from hospital employees can lead to many organizational problems, including morale problems, employee frustration, burnout, and high rates of employee turnover (Ray, 1983; Ray & Miller, 1990; Wandelt, Pierce, & Widdowson, 1981; Wolf, 1981).

Summary

This chapter examined the important and multifaceted role of communication in helping to coordinate the many interdependent groups of people that must work together to accomplish the goals of health care organizations. We analyzed many different aspects of organizational communication in health care. Formal and informal channels of communication were described as the message systems used to connect and inform organization members, clients, and relevant others within the health care system. The importance of coordinating formal and informal communication was clearly emphasized by the first case in the chapter where the formal and informal communication channels of a large hospital were in direct conflict. We examined the development of communication roles and structures in health care organizations, describing some common role conflicts that face members of modern health care systems. We described the growth of bureaucracy in health care organizations and analyzed some of the health care problems associated with the rigidity of bureaucratic systems. The information-processing role of health care organizations was described and illustrated with "The Hospital as an Information System" case history. The interdependent functions of internal and external communication in health care organizations were analyzed. The influences of organizational culture on the coordination of organization members' behaviors were also examined. We concluded the chapter by discussing the role of communication and information in directing organizational development in health care systems, suggesting communication strategies for health care administrators, employees, and consumers to improve the quality of health care systems and health care delivery.

Health Communication Messages and Media

Members of the State Pharmacists' Association were growing more and more concerned with the ability of pharmacists within the state to influence public attitudes about pharmacy and provide the public with accurate information about pharmaceutical products and services. More specifically, they were concerned about poor public recognition of the pharmacist as a health care professional and as an integral member of the health care team, lack of public knowledge about important health care issues, low job satisfaction and self-image of many pharmacists, as well as with public misuse and abuse of medications within the state.

Ernie Floyd, the education director of the Pharmacists' Association

decided, in consultation with the association administrator, that it might
be a good idea for the association to develop a Pharmacists Speakers'
Bureau. He composed a brief questionnaire to survey the reactions
of the association membership about the speakers' bureau idea. Results
of the survey showed that the vast majority of pharmacists who were
members of the association responded positively to the idea of a
speakers' bureau and strongly agreed with the need for improved
information exchange with the public. Paradoxically, very few
pharmacists volunteered to be members of the speakers' bureau and
to make public presentations.

The membership's mixed reaction — they thought the speakers' bureau
was a good idea but were not willing to actively participate in it —
confused Ernie. In the past, the association membership was usually
more than willing to give of their time to participate in activities they
thought to be important. After several discussions with pharmacists,
Ernie discovered the primary reason association members were
reluctant to participate in the program — their lack of confidence in
their ability to speak well in public.

To help pharmacists develop as effective public speakers and to
improve their presentational skills, Ernie arranged a workshop for
association members on presentational speaking. He drafted a
promotional pamphlet about the workshop and sent it out to the
association membership. Local and national experts on public
communication skills training were contacted and arrangements were
made for these experts to lead the workshop. The workshop was
divided into two sessions. The first session was devoted to examining
the public communication process, including preparing the speech,
presenting the speech, and answering audience questions. The second
session was devoted to practicing delivery of public presentations and
used videotape to provide feedback about areas for improvement of
presentational style. Additionally, Ernie put together a speaker
handbook containing tips on public speaking, information on how
to handle questions and answers, how to publicize presentations, how
to find an audience, how to outline a speech, how to utilize audiovisual materials in presentations, where to find information for presentations, and how to critique one's own presentational style.

Attendance at the workshop was good, and it was very successful
at helping the pharmacists apply their expertise to effective
presentational communication. The handbook was distributed to all
workshop participants. After the workshop, several pharmacists
expressed their interest to Ernie in joining the Pharmacy Speakers'

Bureau. The bureau has grown in the months following the workshop, and there are many requests for speakers by different public audiences including schools, churches, senior citizens groups, and business organizations. The speakers' bureau helps to provide these groups with important health information about such varied topics as drug costs, drug abuse, pharmacist services, pharmacy careers, correct uses of medications, vitamins and nutrition, and alcoholism. The Pharmacy Speakers' Bureau is an important part of the State Pharmacists' Association that works to promote better health through health communication. (This case is based on the activities of the Indiana Pharmacist's Association and the work of their director of education, 1981.)

Conveying Information Through Public Communication

Presenting Health Information to the Public

One of the most important aims of health care is to disseminate information which will accurately explain what is happening to the client's body or mind. Conveying information, particularly technical information, is difficult because of differences in language use and cultural systems. It becomes even more challenging to convey health related information to large groups through oral, written, or mediated channels. The purpose of this chapter is to present information that will make it much easier for health and health care information to be shared publicly.

In the case history at the beginning of this chapter, the State Pharmacists' Association used both written and oral communication to develop a Speakers' Bureau. The education director used written communication in preparing a questionnaire to survey the attitudes of pharmacists toward the speakers' bureau, in preparing a brochure promoting the presentational communication workshop, and in preparing the speaker handbook. The presentational communication workshop was presented to the pharmacists through oral communication. Public speaking experts spoke to the pharmacists about public speaking, and the pharmacists then practiced delivering public presentations. As this case history indicates, oral and written presentational communication are important forms of health communication.

Communication and Health Education

One of the most important aims of health care is to disseminate relevant and persuasive health information to those individuals who can best utilize such data to reduce health risks and to increase the effectiveness of health care. This information dissemination/persuasion process is often referred to as health education (Rubinson & Alles, 1984). Both health care consumers and health care providers are important audiences for health education. Consumers need health information to help motivate and direct them to recognize and resist health risks, as well as to seek appropriate treatments for their health problems. Providers need health information to help motivate and direct them to keep up with the latest scientific and clinical findings about health care, enabling them to competently diagnose and treat the different health care problems confronting their clients.

Communication is the primary tool that health educators use in disseminating relevant and persuasive health information. Such communication must be strategic to reach and influence relevant audiences effectively. For example, it is particularly difficult to communicate complex technical information or information that runs counter to established personal and cultural norms (such as persuading heavy smokers to break their habit) due to the unique cultural, educational, and linguistic attributes of different health education audiences. Specific communication strategies must be developed to reach and influence each unique audience. To accomplish their goals, health educators employ a wide range of health communication strategies to adapt to the specific audiences they are addressing and utilize many different communication channels (such as oral, written, and mediated communication) to disseminate relevant health information effectively.

In the case history at the beginning of this chapter Ernie Floyd developed and implemented a health education program designed to teach pharmacists to increase their communication skills as health educators and to motivate them to prepare and present public presentations on relevant health topics. There were two general audiences for health education in this program. The first audience was the pharmacists who needed information and to help them develop health communication strategies and skills. The second audience was consumers of over-the-counter and prescribed pharmaceutical products whom the pharmacists would eventually address about important health care issues as part of the new Pharmacists Speakers' Bureau designed to promote public health education.

Ernie Floyd used both written, oral, and mediated communication strategies to develop and implement the Speaker's Bureau. He used written communication in preparing and administering a questionnaire to survey the attitudes of pharmacists towards the speaker's bureau, in preparing and distributing a brochure promoting the presentational communication workshop, and in preparing and distributing the speaker's handbook. The workshop was presented to the pharmacists with lectures, discussions and feedback sessions using oral communication. Mediated communication was used to present videotape feedback to the pharmacists about their presentational styles and to help them improve their public communication skills. Eventually, when the speaker's bureau is actually implemented, the Pharmacists' Association will disseminate information about the speaker's bureau with posters and pamphlets, as well as with magazine, radio, and television public service announcements and advertisements to attract audiences for their speakers.

In addition to the use of different communication media, health education messages are also disseminated in both *formal* and *informal* communication contexts (Kreps, 1990). Formal health education originates from health care experts and is designed specifically to influence health beliefs, attitudes, and behaviors. For example, health education is presented formally through public presentations about health care issues, health care provider/consumer interactions during office visits, classroom instruction about health care topics, and through mass media programs developed for the specific purpose of disseminating relevant health information. The workshop to help pharmacists develop their speaking skills and the speakers' bureau described in the case at the beginning of this chapter are examples of formal health education.

Informal health education emerges more spontaneously than formal health education. Everyday communication contacts with family, friends, and coworkers provide informal opportunities to discuss health issues. Popular mass media, while not necessarily designed specifically for health education purposes, portray situations which allude to or contain embedded health information. Informal health education can be *directed* and *undirected* (Kreps, 1990). Directed informal health education occurs when people in everyday conversations, who do not have specialized health care training or professional knowledge, offer health care advice. For example, friends or relatives may suggest home remedies for health care problems. Undirected informal health education does not refer specifically to health or health care but contains embedded health information that can influence audiences. Popular magazines, television shows, or films depict the health care behaviors of people or the stories that people tell about health and illness. Many popular stories become cultural legacies in families and communities, leading to the development of culturally based health beliefs and folk remedies. For example, communication of culturally based health care themes concerning the medicinal value of certain foods like chicken soup being "Jewish penicillin," or "an apple a day keeps the doctor away," or "feed a fever, starve a cold" provide the basis for the indoctrination of cultural group members' health beliefs that often guide their health behaviors.

Informal health education performs an important role in helping to establish and maintain culturally approved health care beliefs and practices and is often presented metacommunicatively as a form of cultural socialization. (Recall our earlier discussion of metacommunication as a means for establishing cultural norms in chapter 2.) Informal communication networks are extremely powerful sources of health information since these networks are easily accessible, well-utilized, and personally involving for most people. Unfortunately, there are many instances where the content of health information provided by informal information sources contradicts the most recent and well-documented health care knowledge being disseminated through formal information sources. Popular knowledge about health and health care that contradicts accepted scientific knowledge (such as the unfounded claims of fad diets or oversimplistic folk remedies for complex health care problems) may occasionally be effective in the short-run but often lead individuals to engage in unhealthy long-term health care practices that can harm them and undermine their faith in the formal health care system. For example, the widespread use of untested "underground" drugs and home remedies for AIDS, have often had negative health effects and kept the sick from seeking more established forms of treatment.

Health beliefs strongly influence the health-related behaviors that people choose to perform. The beliefs, values, and attitudes people hold about health and health care color the way these individuals interpret and present health complaints, as well as the way they choose to utilize health information. A member of a religious sect whose culturally induced health beliefs condemn medical technology as evil will react very differently to hospitalization in a modern health care center than will an individual whose health beliefs glorify the development and use of the latest technologies in health care treatment. Health care beliefs inform individuals of the legitimacy of different health care actions and influence their reactions to health information.

Formal and informal health education communicates both content and relationship aspects of health information. (Recall our earlier discussion of content and relationship dimensions of human communication in chapter 2.) Content information in health education concerns descriptive data about the nature of health and health care, while relationship information in health education conveys the level of concern, sensitivity, and power health educators feel towards their audiences. Content and relationship information are interdependent components of health information that must support each other for health education efforts to be successful.

Competent content information in health education communications surrounded by insensitive relationship information will seldom effectively reach and influence its audience. The audience for whom the health education efforts were designed is likely to be insulted and put off by how the health information is being presented. For example, Nancy Reagan's infamously oversimplistic "Just say no," was a message designed to curtail drug abuse and to urge children to reject harmful drugs. However, it failed to recognize the many different situational forces influencing individual drug use and alienated its audience by preaching and speaking down to potential users. Just as problematic as this situation of good health information communicated poorly is bad health information communicated well. Sensitively communicated (good relationship information) health education messages with fallacious health information (poor content information) are very likely to be influential but are unlikely to promote public health. The goal of effective health education then is to provide accurate and relevant health information (good content) using the most appropriate message strategies (relationship information) for the targeted audience.

In actual practice, formal health education efforts are generally most effective at presenting content information and least effective at presenting relationship information. Formal health education, since it is generally offered by knowledgeable health specialists, usually contains timely and accurate health information. Unfortunately, the social distance and, at times, dehumanizing interaction between health care providers and consumers (as well as between health care educators and students) can undermine health education efforts by alienating the recipients of health information.

Paradoxically, informal health education efforts are most effective at presenting relationship information and least effective at presenting content information. Informal health education, since it usually derives from individuals who are not trained health specialists or from those whose primary purpose is not to disseminate health information, often contains unsubstantiated and erroneous health information. Yet, people are usually receptive to informal health education since the information sources are generally comfortable and familiar communication contacts for them. "The public faces a dilemma in using interpersonal sources for health information. Those persons who have the most authoritative information are the least accessible to them. Consequently, the less authoritative but more approachable interpersonal sources are more likely to be used" (Freimuth and Stein, 1987, p. 15). To promote effective interpersonal dissemination of health information, formal health education sources must increase their effectiveness in communicating relationship information, while informal health education sources must increase their abilities to provide accurate and timely content information about health and health care. This can be accomplished in two different ways. First, health care providers and health experts (formal sources of health information) should be trained to communicate health information accurately and sensitively to consumers. Second, public opinion leaders (popular public figures), media hosts (such as Oprah Winfrey), and writers for newspapers, magazines, television, and film (informal sources of health information) should be provided with current and accurate health information and encouraged to disseminate such information.

Oral Dissemination of Health Information

Health care providers and health educators often use public presentations to personally disseminate relevant health information. For these public communication events to be successful, health communicators must communicate strategically. Public communication is much more structured than interpersonal communication. In public communication, one person is usually designated as the presenter and the rest of the participants become the audience. The presenter does the majority of the talking; therefore, the messages presented should be well-organized and persuasive to successfully influence the health beliefs, attitudes, values, and behaviors of audience members.

Public presentations take many forms. Oral presentations can consist of anything from speeches given to laypersons for health education purposes to interprofessional lectures from one health care provider to colleagues for conveying technical information. Obviously, health communicators must analyze the audiences whom they will be addressing to determine the best communication strategies for reaching audience members with their messages. For example, when choosing words to be used in public presentations (whether spoken or written) it is extremely important to be sure the language used is at a level that the audience is likely to understand (Freimuth, 1979; Ley, 1982). Jargon should be used only if the audience members are familiar with the terminology, and examples should be developed to help audience members identify with the points being made in the presentation.

Audience Analysis

It is important to analyze the person or persons with whom you want to share information. The process of doing this is called *audience analysis*, and it is an important one for the health professional to understand. Audience analysis should be done before doing any speaking or writing. You should ask questions such as the following: Whom are you addressing? What are they like? How do you think they will react to your presentation? For example, are you designing information sheets for the diabetic patient, or are you conveying the results of some new research to the county medical association where the relationship is more collegial and the use of more technical language is appropriate? Whatever the case, you need to think about the persons receiving the information. No matter how many people there are (1 or 100), they are your audience. The health professional should analyze the audience members according to such demographic variables as age, education, sex, socioeconomic status, emotional maturity, and the desire to know or understand what is happening to their health in order to determine their cultural orientations and potential attitudes toward you and your topic.

Oral Presentations

It is important to determine the attitude the audience will have toward you and the information you will be presenting. Are you trying to convey information and gain good will? Even though you may be an expert, do the persons you are addressing recognize your expertise, or is it necessary to convince them? All of these questions refer to your credibility. In the broadest sense, *credibility* refers to an audience's willingness to trust what a person says or does. Your manner and presentation will need to be tailored according to the audience's perception of your credibility. Additional audience analysis questions that you should ask when making an oral presentation are: How will the audience arrive at your presentation? Will they be tired from other activities? Are they dreading this speech or anxious to hear it? Is the audience composed of laypersons or experts? Is it a mix? How many will attend?

Regardless of how you answer these and other audience analysis questions, it is important to think about what you want the audience to learn. Although speeches can be designed to inform, to stimulate, and to entertain, all have at least a minimal persuadability component. That is, the speaker is trying to influence the attitudes, feelings, or behaviors of the members of the audience. We will discuss persuasion in a later part of this chapter.

After you have analyzed the audience, you will want to look at your own motives for giving the speech. Do you have important information you want to share with this group to enhance the health of your listeners? Do you want to enhance your reputation as an expert? In answering this latter question, don't be modest. All of us like to share our knowledge in some way or another. We simply need to be honest about our motive.

There are several different types and purposes of public presentations. There are speeches to inform, speeches to persuade, and speeches to entertain. Speeches to inform may include in-service lectures, patient demonstrations, and client health education talks. Speeches to persuade may include fund-raising talks, medical supplies and equipment sales pitches, as well as talks to health consumers and their families to promote compliance with health care regimens. Speeches to entertain may include after dinner presentations at banquets, awards ceremonies, and humorous roasts of colleagues.

Modern speech theorists recognize that most public presentations combine elements of all three of these speech types: information, persuasion, and entertainment. For example, in a good health education lecture, although the primary purpose of the speaker is to inform the audience about a particular health care topic, the speaker also wants to persuade and entertain the audience. The effective speaker attempts to persuade the audience to accept and adopt the point of view given in the presentation and not merely hear the information presented. The effective speaker also wants to make the presentation entertaining and engaging enough to keep the audience's attention and leave them feeling good about the lecture. The best speakers are those who combine the abilities to present clear, relevant information to an audience, to persuade and motivate the audience to respond, and to keep the audience's interest.

Before making a speech, you should analyze your purposes for making the presentation and analyze the audience to whom you are speaking. This prior analysis will help you prepare your presentation because it will provide you with a clear understanding of what you want to do and whom you want to address.

Content and Organization of Speeches

Once the general audience characteristics are known and the motives and goals are established, the speech can be tailored to fit the needs of the group. We have found the phrase "C.O.D." to be helpful. The letters stand for the content, organization, and delivery which are the major elements of either speeches or lectures (Haakenson, 1977).

Usually a topic has been preassigned for most speeches. It is important that the speaker decide on either a narrow or general interpretation of that topic. For example, if the topic is death and dying, the presenter might want to focus on that topic in general or, more specifically, on death and dying in the hospital context. The decision should be made according to audience needs and time constraints. The topic will come into perspective during the presentation stages as notes are prepared and as the speaker reflects on the message to be given.

Haakenson suggests the following four standards for choosing material about your topic.

1. Material should be relevant. It should amplify the point being made.
2. It should be accurate.

3. It should be of interest and capture the listeners' attention.

4. It should be adequate and not overlong.

Haakenson (1977) gives us a religious illustration to support that premise: A veteran pastor was asked by his new assistant, "How long should I preach when I give my first sermon next Sunday?" "That's up to you," came the reply, "but we feel we don't save any souls after twenty minutes" (p. 208).

Once the main premises of the speech are developed, the speaker needs to develop illustrations for these premises — case histories, examples, statistics, humor, quotations, and audiovisual aids are all examples of supporting data. These data can come from personal experience, research and reading, or information obtained from others.

Important information (key points) for the audience needs to be replicated and reinforced so that these points will be remembered. It has been suggested by some researchers that this replication of relevant facts should take place utilizing a different sensory modality (Bandler and Grinder, 1975). For example, if the point is originally made orally to the listener, it should be reemphasized visually. If the purpose is to tell the audience how much damage is done to the lungs by smoking, a slide of a polluted lung might be used as a visual aid to reemphasize that information.

The actual speech itself should have a central idea with major supporting points. The points should be supported by examples. We have included a speech outline which can be adapted to different kinds of speeches (see Figure 6.1). In preparing a speech, the writer should also remember that the organization can be based on chronological or time sequences. Additionally, it can be logically or topically organized.

As the major ideas are tied together in some kind of sequence, transitions become important. The transitions need to tie part-to-part and part-to-whole. Transitions can be made through enumeration ("Secondly, in assessing your smoking behavior you should keep a daily record") or through summarization. Occasional summaries are often an effective way to make the speech clearer to the audience.

As the speech is organized, persuasive devices should be included where appropriate, particularly if a different kind of health behavior is to be encouraged. The motivational process can be briefly summarized. An effective speaker needs to:

1. Secure attention
2. State a problem or need
3. Offer a solution
4. Help the audience visualize the desirability of the solution
5. Invite definite action

Figure 6.1 Skeleton Outline for a Speech To Stimulate a Change in Behavior

---

Technical Plot	How To Stop Smoking
Introduction	I. Secure the attention of the audience and establish a friendly feeling between yourself and the audience; the most common type of beginning is to relate an incident that can be tied with the behavior you will advocate.
Body Statement of importance of behavior Motive Appeal: Pride	II. Taking the lead from the incident you used in the introduction, point out the desirability for and importance of the behavior change.
Examples	A. Using examples, create a vivid picture of what happens when you smoke. 1. Use personal experiences. 2. Use narration and historical cases. B. Reinforce the importance of not smoking through the startling facts which are quoted from prestigious sources.
Anecdote Quotation Example Instance Instance	1. Keep interest and attention high by using stories and other materials that focus on the importance of this behavior change. 2. Show a *general acceptance* of the behavior and of its desirability by society in general and by the kind of people in this audience. C. Adapt to this immediate audience by narrowing your examples and other supporting materials to show that the behavior is also important to them.
Example Story	1. Use examples involving people like those in the audience. 2. Touch the feelings and emotions of the members of this audience. 3. Make the appeal close to the audience; make certain that the behavior is of real significance to them.
Statement of Behavior	D. Make a transition to a specific statement of the the behavior (not smoking) that the audience is to intensify, suggesting some specific procedure to quit smoking.
Slogan	1. Use some novel device such as alliteration or a slogan to express and to impress the plan on the minds of the audience.
Explanation	2. State in a positive way, without sounding argumentative, what you would like the audience to do.
Conclusion	III. Picture life as it will be when the audience has adopted the behavior—not smoking—and heighten the

desirability in their own minds of doing what you suggest.
A. Here you can afford a bit of mild exaggeration, since everyone should be with you and some overstatement will seem natural.

Example

B. Avoid the abstract—be vivid, concrete—making the picture lively and realistic.
C. Fill in the speech with imagery, illustration, and narration.
D. Start with a rapid restatement of the behavior; add a quotation that vividly suggests a personal commitment on the part of the audience to do as you ask; end with a challenge

---

This outline was adapted from *Instructional Supplement With A Handbook of Communication Exercises: Communication Probes*, B. Peterson and R. W. Pace, Chicago, Science Research Associates, Inc. 1977, p. 82.

Part of the motivation process is, of course, to seek change. Since most people either desire or fear change, the speaker or lecturer needs to be aware of how the audience views the particular change. Strategy then needs to be designed to meet the audience's particular needs for the change contemplated by the speaker. Several specific ideas about the process of persuading an audience follow.

1. Persuasion, part of motivation, is accomplished in many ways. Persuasion can be accomplished through the writer's or speaker's reputation. To enforce your reputation (particularly when you are first building one) you should be forceful and knowledgeable. Additionally, you should use supporting materials that are clear, relevant, and innovative.

2. Persuasion also takes place through emotion. People respond to certain words or ideas in a similar manner. You can appeal to the emotions of the audience by knowing the audience's attitudes.

3. Persuasion can also be accomplished through logic or reason. Using valid evidence and sound reasoning assists in this regard.

Audiovisual Aids

Movie or overhead projectors, graphs and charts, tape or phonograph recordings, or an easel are sometimes useful tools for the speaker. Each aid utilized must meet certain criteria, however, or it should not be utilized. These criteria are:

1. *The aid should be important to the speech.* It should specifically amplify the point being made in the speech. It should not be distracting.
2. *The aid should be seen only as an assisting device.* The point being made should stand without an aid but be better because of it.
3. *Aids should be visible, audible, and in working order.*

The final aspect of the third criterion, "working order," is often a major problem when using audiovisual aids. Can you count the number of events you have attended where the projector broke, didn't focus, or the plug to the overhead didn't fit in the wall? Murphy's law of "whatever can go wrong, will go wrong," seems to apply to the use of audiovisual aids. One invaluable rule is to check out the equipment before you decide to use it and once again just before the presentation. You should practice the speech with the aids in the very area in which the speech is to take place, whenever possible.

Aids should be simple and clear. Complicated displays can distract the audience from the major points being made. If the aid is not neat and clear, the audience will start worrying about the speaker's credibility.

The handout is often used as an aid in medically related presentations. While it can be invaluable in presenting detailed and complex material or in summarizing the presentation, care should be taken in handing it out before the speech. Often it will distract the audience. One exception to this is an outline which, when given at the beginning of a complex presentation, can simplify information for the listener.

Introduction, Body, and Conclusion

Generally, there should always be three discrete sections to every public presentation — the introduction, the body, and the conclusion. Each of these sections performs a different and important function in the oral presentation.

The *introduction* is where the speaker identifies him or herself and sets the topics and goals of the presentation to the audience. Introductions are used to orient the audience to the presentation, as well as to establish audience interest and attention. A good approach for establishing attention is to relate the topic of the presentation to the specific goals or backgrounds of the audience members. Credibility can be established in the introduction section of the presentation by demonstrating the source of your expertise, your trustworthiness (or pure motives for the presentation), and your charisma.

The *body* of the presentation is where the data and evidence for your topic is exhibited to the audience. Statistics, quotations, personal testimony, stories, and examples are often used in the body of the presentation to illustrate the major points of the speech. The body of the presentation should reinforce the goals set for the presentation in the introduction, explicating fully the reasons for these goals and providing the audience with information supporting your primary topic. In most speeches, the body is the longest part of the presentation.

The *conclusion* section of the presentation is used to summarize and amplify the primary points of the presentation. The main topics should be restated in the conclusion in a clear and dramatic manner, thus driving these points home to the audience. If you want the audience to act upon any of the information you have provided them, you must forcefully identify specific actions the members of the audience can take. Be sure to offer recommendations that the audience has the potential to accomplish, explaining how and why they should do what you are asking of them. For example, if you are suggesting that each member of your audience be on their guard against hypertension, it would behoove you to explain why that is important and specify how and where they can have their blood pressure checked. The more specific your concluding suggestions are, the more likely it is that your audience will follow your advice.

The introduction, body, and conclusion sections of your presentation provide your speech with structure and direction. The introduction sets up the topic of your presentation for the audience. The body is used to explicate the main points of your speech and provides the supporting evidence for your position. The conclusion is used to tie the main points of your presentation together and leave the audience with a sense of closure and direction.

Delivery of Oral Presentations

Once the content of the speech is established and well-organized, the delivery aspects should be analyzed. This area includes the speaker's psychological set (happy, sad, or firm), bodily expressions (nonverbal communication), and verbal characteristics (voice, articulation, and language).

First and foremost, speeches need to be delivered with excitement, animation, and enthusiasm. Even topics that are highly technical can be made more interesting by the speaker's own interest in his or her presentation.

The nonverbal communication is also important. Gestures need to flow rather than be rigid. The speaker's physical stance (how she or he holds her or his body) has impact on the audience. One of the more common unconscious problems of many public speakers is the failure to keep both feet on the ground while speaking. Appearance is also part of the nonverbal communication, and clothes should be chosen for the speech according to the image the speaker wants to convey. Eye contact and facial expressions are factors. Make sure that you have eye contact with all members of the audience and that your face expresses your enthusiasm for your topic.

The speaker also needs to think about his or her voice and how it affects the audience. Can they be heard in the back of the room? One trick is to always project the voice to the person in the furthermost corner. The pitch of the voice also needs to be considered. The voice should be neither too high nor too low. Additionally, the speaker needs to change inflection once in a while during the speech for persuasive purposes.

Words need to be articulated carefully and at the right rate of speech. Fast speeches are ignored and slow speeches are boring. Additionally, the language of the speech should be appropriate and sometimes eloquent or dynamic. Words such as "uh" and "okay" should be avoided. Again, jargon or "medspeak," as health-related jargon is often called, should be avoided unless the audience will understand the jargon. If the audience consists of laypersons, the speaker should remember the international and national findings which show that patients do not interpret medical terminology in the same way professionals do and care should be taken to avoid such terms (DiMatteo and Freidman, 1982).

Some additional delivery tips include the following:

1. A pause should take place after the speaker stands up. This pause allows organization of notes, a survey of the audience, and a deep breath!

2. Humor can be part of the delivery only if such humor is comfortable for the speaker. Humor should not be forced.

3. The speaker should not apologize for coughing, for forgetting, or for any part of the presentation. In fact, it is very important for him or her to convey an air of confidence about the whole performance.

4. The final portions of the speech or lecture should be effective, persuasive, and enthusiastic. As stated in the content section, a summary is important and the audience should be left thinking about the major points.

5. Speakers should watch other speakers in person and on television for good speaking tips as well as for problems to avoid.

Special Notes on Television Presentations

Television provides invaluable opportunities for health education. However, organization becomes of paramount concern as time is so limited.

Often the health professional will be asked to speak about a broad topic in a limited amount of time — for example, to spend three minutes giving a full analysis of the pros and cons of dairy products. Obviously, there is far more information about this topic than the three-minute limit permits. In preparing for a thirty minute television presentation, the speaker should think of no more than three major points to convey, and the rest of the time should be used in supporting those points. In preparing for talk show presentations (and the preparation takes place with the moderator for five minutes before the camera rolls), the speaker should emphasize the issues he or she thinks will be important to the audience. Talk show hosts or hostesses rarely know the subject as well as the speaker, and often have no idea of the questions to begin asking about technical subjects.

Some ideas for television presentations are:

1. Wear a dark suit or jacket with some contrast in a shirt or blouse. Make sure your clothes aren't too busy.

2. Look at the host or the other panelists. Don't stare into the camera!

3. Watch your feet. Place them firmly on the ground and sit with your back touching the back of your chair. Don't be too rigid or too relaxed.

4. Try to forget you are on television. Talk with the other participants as you would talk with colleagues or friends.

5. Be enthusiastic about your topic.

6. Don't be long-winded. Answers to questions and comments should be forceful but short. Use examples or cases to support your points when possible.

7. Don't be late. Live TV shows can't wait for you. Additionally, make sure you know the studio location in advance. Many of them are hidden in remote areas.

8. Be sure to tell your family and friends to view your performance and to offer suggestions. If you want to assess your own performance, videotape the session.

Notes on Lecturing and Teaching

The lecture is a very important communication tool in health care education. There has been much criticism recently of medical and nursing school teaching. The criticism focuses on such issues as boring lectures, professors' lack of interest in students, and little attention to feedback from the students. Once again, we want to stress that all oral presentations contain elements of speeches to inform, persuade, and entertain. This is especially true of the lecture. A good lecture should do more than merely present information to an audience. The lecture should be designed to present pertinent information, motivate the audience to accept and use the information, and keep the audience involved and interested in the lecture.

It should be noted that the word *doctor* is derived from the Latin word *docere* meaning "to teach." Teaching is an essential part of health care practice, as it is an essential part of both providing consumers with relevant health care information and training health care professionals about the latest health care methods. While efforts have been made to improve health-related teaching by adding "teachers of teachers" to several medical and nursing school faculties, recent cutbacks in the funding of these programs have eliminated some of these programs which focus on good teaching. In an attempt to facilitate increased recognition of the importance of oral communication in teaching, as well as the abilities to communicate effectively in teaching situations, we suggest a few teaching tips.

The lecture needs to contain interesting and stimulating material, be pertinent to the specific audience, and be well-organized and well-delivered. The use of humor, case studies, and other devices can be effective in emphasizing important points. Handouts are often useful for presenting highly technical or complex material.

The major difference between the lecture and most public presentations is in the area of feedback from the audience. In most public presentations, there is a specific time period set aside for questions and answers. During a lecture, however, students generally need to ask questions and, at times, engage in discussion. Often these interchanges can divert the class and the teacher from the lecture topic. An effective lecturer needs to be flexible enough to deal with student concerns while tying class interaction to the lecture topic and meeting the time demands of the class period. The lecturer should attempt to make transitions between the comments students make and the lecture topic being presented. In this way, the lecturer is able to answer the questions and respond to the audience's ideas while keeping the presentation on topic. Additionally, allowing time for questions during or after the lecture can help the lecturer keep track of the topic and make the presentation within the given time limits.

Research on the attention span of audiences and our personal experiences as educators suggest that lectures can reach a point of diminishing return for the speaker if they are too long. Generally, the lecturer should not speak to an audience on a complex topic for more than forty-five minutes at a stretch if students are expected to retain material (Harlem, 1977). It is a good idea to break up long lectures with question and answer sessions, illustrations, exhibits, media, group exercises, or group discussions to keep your audience's attention.

An important technique for teachers (as well as for other speakers) is to seek feedback from students as well as to answer questions. In seeking feedback, the lecturer can find out if students are understanding the material, and if they think the lecturer is effective. Those of us who have taught know how difficult it is to accept this feedback. However, if students are to learn, we certainly need to ascertain the effectiveness of our teaching.

Lectures to one's colleagues follow much the same format as to students; however, they can be more technical. For special information on this topic Calnan and Barabas (1972) have designed a useful guide in their short book, *Speaking at Medical Meetings.* Although this book is directed toward physicians, it is also useful for those in other health care professions.

Public communication often overlaps with group communication. In formal group situations, the group leader and selected group members may find themselves in the position of addressing the group. These presentations to groups contain many of the same characteristics of speeches that have been discussed in this chapter. Chapter 4 examined the topic of communication in groups.

Written Communication

Conveying Public Information

Both the oral and the written word are important to the health professional. As we have discussed, the setting, the audience, and the time are some of the factors that influence whether information should be shared orally or in writing. Speeches are usually more informal. Oral language must be understood immediately; it is more difficult to replicate information orally. The speaker has an opportunity to gain feedback, particularly in informal settings; it is much more difficult for the writer to achieve that dialogic component.

The reasons that writing is chosen over speaking, however, are many. Sometimes writing is a reinforcement to speaking. For example, a physician might prescribe medication, giving the patient oral instructions, and then choose to replicate with the new written information sheets provided by the American Medical Association in its Patient Medication Instruction Program. The physician might also choose to design his or her own information sheets. Writing is also important if the health care professional wants to reach large numbers of people. Writing often reaches a larger audience because it is easier to disseminate written materials, and people can view these materials at their own leisure, in their own home environment.

It is also considered academically and scientifically important that many health professionals "publish" at some time in their careers (Harlem, 1977). The written word is an important means of time-binding knowledge across generations. Writing is considered particularly credible for the researcher because the written document allows scrutiny by one's peers. Types of health or medically related writings are prescriptions, written patient instructions, technical-research papers, case reports, and patient records. The health professional might also choose to write poetry or publish both fiction and nonfictionalized accounts of health care.

One serious concern that faces the writer of information-sharing technical papers is the long period of time from the generation of a research idea to the date of publication of the results. Often painstaking research work becomes outdated before it is published. The prospective writer needs to be aware of the lengthy process of article submission, review, and actual publication. Publication sources should be chosen accordingly.

Anyone considering serious writing of any kind should be clear about their motives. Are they writing for professional advancement and/or recognition by their peers? Are they writing to share data with their colleagues that might assist patient care? Are they writing because they have a creative urge? Being clear about one's motives is important because it helps guide the direction of the written work.

The second important question is "What do you want to write?" After the first goal question is answered, the answer to this second question becomes clearer. For example, if you are writing for national recognition from colleagues, you might want to write a carefully structured and somewhat original article or letter to a national journal. Research might be presented in several ways: orally at a specific convention and in written form to specific or more generalized audiences. Some professional associations have combined both goals by publishing oral presentations in written form in a proceedings format.

The third question, "What audience do you want to address in your writing?" ties into the other questions. By deciding what you want to write, you usually demarcate a possible audience. If you are a nurse practitioner wanting to share some carefully constructed case studies, you need to find the appropriate journal. If you are a pharmaceutical researcher, your audience will usually read pharmacy journals.

Content and Organization of Writing

In the early part of this chapter, we advocated the "Content-Organization-Delivery" method of speech organization. That method is equally applicable to writing. In this section we will apply that method to the writing of a research report. Case studies will also be mentioned.

The *title* is important because it indicates not only what the subject material is, but where it will be filed in abstracts and indices. It is important that the title encapsulate the paper. Usually, the title is followed by an *abstract* which is a summary or overview of the entire research endeavor. The abstract gives the reader an opportunity to decide whether he or she wants to read the entire report and should be comprehensive and stimulating.

The *introduction* to the report gives justification for the research. It is this paragraph or paragraphs that are the most difficult to write. Rather than agonize over this first paragraph or sentence, we encourage the author to put anything down just to get started. In fact, this first paragraph can more easily be made consistent with the paper after the paper is complete. These first paragraphs should also incorporate the research goal which, of course, should have been established before the research was started.

Failure to delineate the problem clearly in the introduction reflects on the research as well as the writer's ability to think clearly. However, once again, rather than agonize over the appropriate words at this stage of writing, a raw statement of the purpose can be temporarily put on paper so that the writer can move ahead to the body of the paper which is usually the easiest part of the paper to write. An example of a first paragraph follows:

> The purpose of the study was to investigate correlations between human and animal infanticide. It was hypothesized that the instinctual drive that leads to baby killing in animals may have a counterpart in humans which leads to child abuse and maltreatment.*

Related research is usually discussed at the beginning of the research report, after the statement has been clearly presented. In this section of the report the author summarizes the relevant research of others and gives the citations of those research reports so that the reader can look them up if necessary. This is generally one of the easiest sections of the paper to write since it is simply a compilation of the data of others. It is important in this section of the report to summarize and quote accurately.

The *method and design* of the research are presented next. The writer needs to explain what method was used (experimental? historical? descriptive?) and how it was used. It is in this section of the report that a description of the subjects and the methods employed is pertinent. Ethical considerations and safeguards should also be noted.

In the *results* section of the report, the researcher sets forth the

---

*This was adapted from a news story on animal infanticide research. *Nevada State Journal*, October 26, 1982.

interpretations of the data. If the research utilized hypotheses, this is the time to state whether those hypotheses were rejected or accepted according to the data analysis.

The last part of the paper centers around a discussion of the research. A summary is included at this point and the resolution of the initial research problems is discussed. Conclusions are stated here as well as applicability to specific situations. Suggestions for future research based on the study can be discussed at this point. *Notes and references* follow the body of the paper. It is important that every quote as well as all other material utilized directly from other sources be properly identified.

Examples of research papers and technical reports which are medically oriented can be found by looking at major index sources (see Figure 6.2).

Figure 6.2   Selected Health and Medicine Indices

Abstracts of Health Care Management Studies: Includes articles on general health care. Abstracts are given.

Hospital Literature Index: This index offers material related to hospitals and health care in many types of facilities.

Index Medicus: This is probably the major index focusing on health related subjects. It includes subject and author sections. Journals indexed are found in the January issue. It does not abstract.

International Nursing Index: Has subject and author sections and each topic is indexed under at least three headings. Journals are in the January issue. The index also has publications of organizations and agencies as well as authors.

Medical Socioeconomic Resource Source: This is designed to integrate material from social science and the health care field. Economic and public health are two of the fields indexed. It does contain brief abstracts.

Newsbank: A newspaper clipping service not available in all libraries. Indexes articles from over 100 cities. Topics are included from socioeconomic, political, and scientific fields.

Hospital Literature Index: This index offers material related to hospitals and health care in many types of facilities.

The Case Study Report

In recent years, the case study report has often been deemphasized while laboratory studies have been more prominent in the medical journals. Medicine and health, however, can often be better understood and health practice methods can be shared if the case study is utilized. It is also a good starting point for medical writers (Harlem, 1977). Case studies need to be presented carefully and should be somewhat unusual so that the material will be useful to the reader. The writer of the case study report, in conjunction with any technical writer, needs to research his or her subject well to make sure that identical case presentations do not already exist in the literature; if they do exist, this new presentation must bring new and thoughtful ideas. The writer also needs to find a suitable journal which encourages case studies. In other words, the writer needs to find the right audience. Once again, Figure 6.2 needs to be consulted for major health and medically related index sources. These sources list the major publications of the many health fields in addition to providing information on research reports in the journals. Another important advantage of the case study report is that it gives private practitioners a conduit to their academic colleagues. Harlem (1977) emphasizes the fact that private practioners are not part of the "in-group" that writes articles for medical journals although they have much to offer the practice of medicine. He suggests that writing cases is one way to improve communication between academicians and practitioners. His ideas on this would apply to any health care field.

Delivery or Presentation of Written Communication

Though the term delivery is usually associated with public speaking, we argue that it needs to be considered as equally important to written communication. The delivery or presentational aspects of the material often determine whether the document will be read or not. A paper, a book, or even an instruction sheet to a client needs to be neat and pleasing to the eye. The typing or printing of the document should be done carefully with no errors. Headings should draw the reader's attention. Pages should be carefully numbered.

Additionally, the document should not be too lengthy. Unless it is full of highly important technical data which a specialized audience will read, major points and summaries should be stressed with citations included for anyone who wants to do further research. Put yourself in the place of one of your anticipated readers and ask if you would read the document you have prepared. This question, more than any other, will assist you in preparing your manuscript or document for delivery to a publisher or audience.

Turning Speeches into Written Papers

There is a desire common to many writers to turn oral presentations into written papers which can be submitted for publication. Unfortunately, this is not as easy as it sounds. Words that appeal during a speech are often too informal to be committed to paper. While speech making requires some color and warmth, technical papers require more formal and remote presentations. Points made in writing are longer and more complex. While the same formula can be used for either speeches or writing (content, organization, and delivery), the ways words are presented in the different speaking or writing contexts must be evaluated differently by the speaker-writer. Reworking the speech with these considerations in mind can often solve the problem. Sometimes, however, a new outline needs to be developed with more attention given to examples suitable for writing as well as to charts and visual aids more appropriate for a paper than a speech.

Instruction Sheets

The relatively recent finding that it is important to repeat information to clients is beginning to penetrate medicine and health care. The physician, or nurse, or other health educator is often called upon to take highly technical information and reduce it orally and in writing so that the client can understand and follow a regimen. The challenge becomes particularly acute in instruction sheets where the information needs to be condensed to one or two pages. Nowhere is content, organization, and delivery such a challenge. Avoiding "medspeak" (the jargon health professionals, particularly physicians, use to share information) and asking clients to review the material before it is printed are two important tips. In a study on communication with clients, it was found that 81 percent of the physicians underestimated their clients' capabilities to understand explanations. The study found that clients actually were able to understand most problems if they were discussed in ordinary language (DiMatteo-Friedman, 1982).

In writing instruction sheets, points can be underlined and enumerated (1, 2, 3, 4, etc.) to indicate their importance. Headings are also important on short documents.

Letters

Health care practitioners who have little time but much to say are often found writing letters to editors. *The New England Journal of Medicine* is noted for the dialogue that takes place through letters on major health issues. The letter-writing sections of journals provide a democratic forum for an exchange of ideas among colleagues as well as among members of other professions.

Such communications should be written on standard business paper and should follow a business letter form. They should follow some logic, be brief, and be to the point. Even if disagreement is being expressed, the letter is usually more effective if it relies on facts and logic rather than on a passionate subjective opinion. Letters sometimes need to be written to colleagues and clients. Neatness, clarity, and a direct approach to the subject are the cornerstones of an effective business letter. The presentation and delivery are also of importance. Impressive printed stationary and no typographical errors are examples of the latter.

Seeking Reaction from Others

One of the most important steps in writing of any kind is to have your work reviewed and edited informally before it is submitted to official reviewers. This is not an easy thing to accomplish. Friends and family members are sometimes too complimentary or too critical. The person or persons who are seeking to review your work informally should be persons who have some knowledge of your subject. Ideally, the reviewer should represent the audience you are seeking through your writing. The copy of your material to be reviewed should be widely spaced and contain plenty of room for margin writing. Ask the reader to correct misspellings, to mark awkward sentences, and to comment on the readability and accuracy of your writing. Be sure to indicate a time frame for the criticism. Most importantly, put yourself in a state of mind which allows you to look forward to the criticism, knowing that it will make a better final product. Don't be defensive with your informal review. Take all criticism given but decide for yourself what changes need to be made in your writing. At this point, put yourself in the place of your audience.

Mediated Communication and Health Information

Modern societies have become increasingly dependent upon media to disseminate health information, enabling the sharing of relevant health information among many different people, groups, and organizations within modern societies (Atkin & Wallack, 1990). Media provide forums for information that help societal members recognize and evaluate environmental opportunities and constraints, coordinate their resources and activities in response to their environment, learn about culturally relevant phenomena, and pass on (time-bind) knowledge and cultural information to future societies as a form of social inheritance (Kreps, 1988). Mediated communication is often used in public health education campaigns by channelling health information to consumers about health promoting behaviors (Atkin & Wallack, 1990; Flay & Cook, 1981). For example, mediated communication has been used, with differing levels of success, to provide consumers with information about the uses and abuses of drugs (Flay, 1986), the importance of good nutrition (Kaufmen, 1980; Ivy & Stokes, 1987), how to avoid heart disease (Maccoby & Farquhar, 1975; Maccoby & Solomon, 1981; Solomon, 1984), preventing drunk driving (Atkin, Garramone, & Anderson, 1986), the importance of giving up smoking (Bauman, Brown, Bryan, Fisher, Padgett, & Sweeney, 1989; Flay, 1987), and reasons and methods for effective contraception (Schellstede & Ciszewski, 1984; Udry, 1972).

McLuhan (1964) describes media as the "extensions of man." The use of media extends people's ability to communicate, to speak to others far away, to hear messages, and to see images that would be unavailable without media. As extensions to human communication, media allow health care professionals to reach more people with health related messages in less time than through nonmediated communication channels. Media enable people who are geographically removed from health care organizations and personnel to access health care information without traveling long distances. Media have been used as a powerful educational tool, serving a wide range of audiences, including students of the health sciences, practicing health care professionals, and health care consumers. Later in this chapter we present a case history which describes a real situation where videotape was used as an in-house tool in an urban hospital for providing health care consumers with relevant information. Media provide powerful tools for storing and transmitting important health care information. Modern health care services depend upon the use of media as communication tools, and these uses and applications of mediated communication in the delivery of health care will continue to expand in the future.

Media are tools that people use to communicate ideas and information. A definition of media follows: *media are an intermediary communication delivery system using some form of technology.* By an intermediary system, we mean media are used as a specialized channel of communication between communicators. Different kinds of media technologies have been developed to link communicators. These include print, audio, video, and computer technologies. Some of these media are designed to appeal to the general public. The public channels of mediated communication are known as *mass media.* Other forms of media are designed for use with selected groups of people, usually within the boundaries of organizations. These private channels of mediated communication are generally known as *in-house media.* In this chapter, we will explore a wide range of applications and implications of mass media and in-house media on the delivery of health care.

In discussing mediated communication, we will distinguish among three broad types of media, each possessing various different specialized media tools. The three broad types of media are: *print media, audiovisual media,* and *interactive media.*

Print Media

Print media, such as newspapers, books, magazines, journals, and pamphlets, are the oldest and most traditional of the three forms of mediated communication we will examine in this chapter. They have great utility as health communication tools to educate consumers about health risks, health maintenance, and health care services (Atkin & Wallack, 1990). Print media rely on the use of the written word, incorporating both photography and sophisticated graphic designs. Such media are used both as in-house communication channels in health care delivery systems (such as hospitals) as well as communication channels to reach larger audiences. To reach specialized audiences health care systems typically use employee newsletters, annual reports, letters, booklets, bulletin boards, posters, payroll inserts, handbooks, company magazines, and exhibits. To reach more general audiences books, newspapers, magazines, and billboards are often used. It is critical that these print media be written clearly (at an appropriate level) and engagingly for the audiences for which they are intended.

Newspapers are one of the most widespread forms of print media. Most of us are exposed to newspapers daily. Newspapers strongly influence public beliefs, attitudes, and behaviors by setting the agenda for what their readers think about (Cohen, 1963; McCombs & Shaw, 1972). Yet, the press has had a much greater influence on political campaigns than it has had on public health campaigns, perhaps due to the limited amount of space devoted to health issues (Sobel & Brown, 1982; Wallack, 1981). The ability of the press to influence public health behaviors should increase now as both the amount of space given to these issues and the sophistication of health writing appears to be increasing (Brown & Einsiedel, 1990; Wallack, 1990).

Interestingly, Wright (1975) found in a survey of the comparative use of newspapers, radio, magazines, and television as sources of health information, that newspapers and magazines were used most often by respondents and printed media were identified as the most useful source of health information. Bishop (1974) found that the more pious consumers are about a specific health problem, the more likely they are to seek and utilize printed health information. Pamphlets and booklets are examples of technologically simple, but important, print media used by many health care systems to provide their relevant publics with health information (Feldman, 1966). These print media are often used to help consumers recognize and understand symptoms of health problems, adopt appropriate strategies for resisting and coping with health risks, and identify where and how they can obtain health care services.

Print media, specifically biomedical journals and textbooks, have been found to be an important and preferred source of health information for health care providers, helping them learn about the latest techniques for diagnosing and treating health problems (Covell, et al., 1985; Currie, 1976; Stinson & Mueller, 1980). Yet, advances in health care knowledge are expanding at such a rapid rate that it is increasingly difficult for health care providers who depend upon state-of-the-art health information to keep up-to-date (Bernier & Yerkey, 1979; Harlem, 1977; Haynes, et al., 1986; Kreps, Hubbard, & DeVita, 1988). Bernier and Yerkey (1979) estimated that approximately two million articles are published in the biomedical literature annually and the publication rate was increasing geometrically, making it virtually impossible for health care providers to keep abreast of the relevant literature on health care advances. In fact, evidence suggests that the longer it has been since most physicians have graduated from medical school, the more outdated their health care knowledge and practices become (Haynes, et al., 1986). Medical abstracting services that provide brief summaries of pertinent literature help health care providers cope with the information overload created by the rapidly expanding body of health literature, as do the publication of scientific review articles that summarize and critique bodies of literature. Later in this chapter we will discuss the use of computerized databases to help people cope with the ever-expanding volume of health information.

Audiovisual Media

Audiovisual media are a powerful form of communication that use recording technologies to dramatically present sounds and sights to audiences in such forms as radio, television, and film. Commercial radio and television are particularly important channels for disseminating health information. Radio and television have become increasingly health oriented in recent years, with increased programming of shows and stories concerning health issues (Gerbner, Gross, Morgan, & Signorielli, 1981; Signorielli, 1990; Turow, 1989). For example, news programs often include special "health sense" and even employ "health reporters." Nationally televised news magazine shows, such as "60 Minutes," "20-20," and "Hour Magazine," generally offer special segments devoted to health issues such as nutrition, heart disease, exercise, and new health care treatments. Discussion-oriented television shows, such as "Donahue," often invite nationally recognized health experts or individuals with life-threatening health problems to interact with a live audience about health topics. Exercise shows provide their audience with health-promoting ideas and activities. Radio talk shows often discuss health issues and provide listeners with health care tips. To the extent that the health information presented via these media is valid, the health programming trends have helped make television and radio important channels for health promotion.

Unfortunately, information presented through mass media do not always promote public health. For example, advertisements for cigarettes and alcoholic beverages have downplayed the health risks associated with these products, implied that consumption of these products enhances virility, athleticism, and sophistication, and are often directed toward high-risk segments of the population, such as youths who may develop hard-to-break negative health habits early in their lives (Jacobson & Amos, 1985; Novelli, 1990; Trauth & Huffman, 1986). Furthermore, dramatic programs on television and popular films often present distorted images of the health care system, commonly representing the health care professional as omnipotent or representing the health care system as inept (McLaughlin, 1975; Signorielli, 1990; Turow, 1989).

Exaggerated media portrayals of the health care system can lend support to inaccurate societal stereotypes about the roles of health care providers and consumers and may promote many unrealistic expectations consumers have of the health care system. Dramatic media programs and advertisements that glorify the use of products associated with serious health risks and present stereotypical portrayals of health care situations can reinforce unrealistic expectations for health and health care practice and encourage the development of unproductive public health beliefs (Kasl & Cobb, 1966; Novelli, 1990). Despite the serious problems of distorted presentations of health and health care by popular media, these audiovisual mass media channels have great potential for use as powerful tools for public health promotion if they are used to provide the public with strategically designed messages concerning relevant health information (Wallack, 1990). (In chapter 9 we will consider several of the strategic message design issues that must be examined to develop effective health promotion media programs.)

Audiovisual media are also commonly used in health care institutions, such as hospitals, as important in-house and public organizational communication tools. Commonly used hospital-based audiovisual media include videotape, film, sound/slide programs, and cassette tapes used for staff and consumer education, reports between shifts, documenting health care procedures (often for legal purposes), health promotion campaigns, as well as for hospital public relations projects (Burge, 1981). Videotape is a powerful audiovisual communication media that has found extensive use in hospitals (Elmore, 1981). Videotape has been successfully used in medical education programs to help physicians develop effective communication skills by recording practice interviews and presentations and by playing the recordings back, providing the physicians with direct feedback about communication performance (Cassata & Clements, 1978). Recall how videotape feedback was used in the Pharmacist Speaker's Bureau training program to help the pharmacists refine their presentational speaking skills.

In addition to video technology, films, slide/sound programs, and audio tapes are also commonly used in many health care organizations for staff and consumer education. Many hospitals maintain their own media libraries where clients and staff can access a broad range of different health care media programs. Many hospitals also maintain their own media production departments that work with health care staff to produce relevant audiovisual media. For example, in the following case history note how the hospital used videotape media to promote health education by producing its own consumer education video program. Why do you think the audiovisual program developed in this case facilitated such a dramatic change in consumer behavior?

St. Francis Hospital of Indianapolis was encountering an unexpected problem. A rather large number of clients at the hospital, whose physicians had recommended that they have a gastroscopy, refused to sign the informed consent statement and would not undergo the procedure. Gastroscopies are fairly routine procedures which involve the use of a gastroscope instrument to inspect the interior of the stomach. The gastroscope, which is a tube-like instrument with something similar to a light on its end, is inserted through the client's mouth, down the esophagus, and into the stomach. The procedure is invaluable in examining ulcers, discovering tumors of the stomach, and generally discovering stomach disease. Although the procedure sounds rather involved and uncomfortable, it is relatively simple and causes most clients very little discomfort. Lack of adequate information from the physician about what the client could expect before, during, and after the procedure was thought to be the problem. After reviewing the situation, including interviews with hospital staff and clients, it was decided that there should be a gastroscopy educational program developed. The hospital media department produced an informative videotape designed to describe the gastroscopy procedure and its uses. The videotape program included interviews with physicians, nurses, and those who were just recovering from the procedure. The videotape program was shown to each hospital client recommended for a gastroscopy. Client response to the media program was extremely positive. The informed consent turn-down rate was reduced by 35 percent for those who watched the brief videotape presentation.

Interactive Media

One of the most interesting and powerful applications of media in health care is the use of *interactive media*, which allow people to send, process, and receive health information through the use of different new communication technologies. Both reflective and intelligent interactive media are used to provide users with relevant health information. *Reflective* media (such as the telephone, closed circuit television, and electronic mail) recreate users' messages for dissemination to other users, while *intelligent* media (such as computerized information, education, and diagnostic systems) interpret user initiated requests for information, process data, and respond with appropriate answers to user requests. The common telephone is an example of a reflective interactive media which enables users to communicate across vast distances by transmitting their vocal and facsimile (FAX) messages. Computer information systems, such as the National Cancer Institute's Physician Data Query (PDQ), are examples of intelligent interactive media which do not merely recreate users' messages, but provide users with answers to specific information requests. The PDQ system provides users with state-of-the-art cancer treatment information for the specific type and stage of cancer about which the user wants to know (Kreps, Hubbard, & DeVita, 1988).

The telephone is an important communication tool that allows people all over the world the potential to interact with one another. Advancements in telecommunications technology have increased the power and flexibility of telephone systems, providing communicators with a variety of special features such as voice mail, call forwarding, call waiting, automatic call back, automatic call out, and teleconferencing functions. Increasingly, the telephone has been utilized as a health information dissemination medium, with telephone mediated hot lines and referral services developing as important channels for providing support, information, and referral for callers who suffer from assorted health risks such as AIDS, poisoning, domestic violence, alcoholism, drug addiction, and cancer. Local and national telephone hot lines provide millions of callers with crisis counseling, helping lonely, depressed, and suicidal callers to work through their emotional problems (Fish, 1990). For example, the National Cancer Institute has developed a cancer information hot line, administered by the Cancer Information Service (CIS), that can be reached by anyone in the United States via a toll-free telephone number (1-800-4-CANCER) for up-to-date information regarding cancer treatment, referral, and clinical research (Freimuth, Stein, & Kean, 1989). The CIS hot line has been used successfully in concert with other communication media such as the PDQ information system to provide callers with relevant health information. The CIS has also successfully used print, radio, and television advertisements and public service announcements to promote the hot line to the public (Freimuth, Stein, & Kean, 1989).

Some of the difficulties inherent in the use of the telephone as a mediated form of communication involve the limitations of the technical channel to hold information and the tendency toward distortion and loss of information between communicators over the telephone. These two problems are closely tied to one another. The obvious limitation of the telephone as a channel of information, as compared to face-to-face interpersonal communication, is the loss of visual, tactile, olfactory, kinesic, proxemic, and artifactic information. The standard telephone used by the public is generally limited to providing users with verbal, paralinguistic, and chronemic information. As we discussed in chapter 2, people use the various different channels of verbal and nonverbal communication messages to confirm and clarify the overall message being sent. They examine the range of messages available to them and decipher the content of the communication situation through a process of comparison and contrast. In chapter 2 we suggested that effective communicators are aware of the range of different messages they send and strive to be perceptive of the various verbal and nonverbal messages others send to them. The telephone limits the range of messages communicators have available to send and receive. This constraint on the number of messages available to communicators increases the opportunities for message distortion in telephone communication situations.

The implications of these limitations on telephone communication serve to introduce several potentially troublesome situations for health communicators. One significant problem posed is the probability of sending and receiving misconstrued messages. The effectiveness of communication in health care often depends on the accuracy of message reception. For example, if a physician misconstrues a lab technician's telephoned report of the results of a lab test by just one decimal point, the resulting incorrect diagnosis or treatment plan enacted can have dangerous repercussions for the client. A second, related, potential problem in telephone communication is the use of the medium for purposeful deception. It is more difficult to detect deception over the telephone than in face-to-face communication due to the limited range of messages the receiver has to interpret. For example, a caller may disguise his or her voice over the phone, without any fear of being recognized by a visual cue. To improve the accuracy of communication over the telephone and limit the occurrence of unintentionally misconstrued or purposefully deceptive messages, communicators must pay close attention to the verbal, paralinguistic, and chronemic messages available to them. Moreover, telephone communicators should utilize feedback to clarify messages sent and received. (See chapter 2 for a discussion of how best to use feedback.) The introduction of telephones with the technical capability of transmitting both audio and video signals (the picture phone) will increase the message sending capacity of the telephone, although it still will not approach the message capacity of face-to-face communication.

Closed circuit television is another interactive communication medium used in health care that is similar to the telephone, yet has the potential for providing users with more message information than the conventional telephone. Interactive television can provide users with both visual and audio message information. This can be essential in health care situations where a health care provider may have to see as well as hear a description of the consumer to effectively diagnose and treat an ailment. Park and Bashshur (1975) have described the use of two-way closed circuit television as "telemedicine," explaining its use as a communication tool for ". . . remote diagnosis, consultation, counseling, psychotherapy, and teaching." They identify several interactive media programs that are being used to provide health care information and services to people via two-way television technology. The consequences of telemedicine for health care providers and health care practice are that health care services formerly unavailable to individuals in remote locations can now be offered via specialized media. Satellites have been developed to provide health communication information via two-way radio and television to remote geographic areas, affording people living in rural areas like "bush" Alaska with the benefits of modern health care information and services.

Computer technology can be used with telephones and closed circuit television media to provide health care organizations with exciting interactive communication capabilities. Computers are powerful cybernetic communication tools that can process information and respond to different user requests. The computer is an intelligent interactive communication technology. When used as an adjunct to the telephone or the closed circuit television system, the computer can be used to rapidly evaluate and analyze incoming off-site information, search distant information banks for solutions to problems, and direct user behavior in accordance with precedents established in external health care facilities. The computer can be used to evaluate the likelihood of success of a given health maintenance procedure, analyze the data produced from many complicated lab tests, or search for related research and evidence upon which to base a health care decision, all in a highly time and cost efficient manner.

A major problem encountered in computer use is the impersonality of many computers and computer programs. The computer is unable to interact on a "human" analogic level, is unable to understand emotions such as fear, anger, frustration, love, and so on, and is seen as being a cold, unfeeling machine by many users. Moreover, most of the programs designed for computers make the computer a very unforgiving communication tool. With these programs a user has to be able to send an absolutely correct entry message to the computer, using the computer's language or code, or the computer will not provide the user with the information or services requested. Minor message inadequacies like a misplaced punctuation mark or a lower case letter entered where a capital letter should be, are enough to jam communication between the user and the computer.

Modern programmers have done their best to rectify the impersonality and rigidness of the computer by designing convivial programs for computer users. Convivial programs often use nontechnical computer languages modeled after human languages and have personalized error messages that playfully identify any syntax problems a user may have presented to the computer. Older nonconvivial computer programs would merely reply to an incorrect user entry with a flashing "ERROR" statement. Newer convivial programs cue the computers to reply in a more friendly manner with a response such as, "Sorry, I think you made a mistake. Here is how to enter your request so I can read it. Thanks a lot!" Additionally, several computer games have been designed that are fun for users to play and make the modern computer a much more enjoyable communication tool than older nonconvivial computers. As computer programmers continue to develop convivial computer systems and as users become more sophisticated about computer methods and applications, the computer will continue to grow as an important form of interactive media in health care.

Computers have been used widely as a form of in-house interactive media. They are used to process both words and numbers for users. Computers have been found to be a handy and efficient means of storing data for future retrieval. Health care organizations depend on computers to store and process their financial data, medical records, personnel information, and inventory of supplies and equipment. Computer users communicate with the computer, using an accepted computer language or code, to access the information the computer has stored. New technologies have enabled computers to share information. That is, given the right access codes, one computer can obtain information stored in another computer, usually through a telephone interface. An organization with a computer and a telephone interface mechanism can access a wide range of information and information processing services.

There are many organizational applications for computer technologies for storing, processing, and retrieving health information in health care systems. Computers are commonly used to store and process medical records, information about health care treatment, referral, and research, as well as to analyze laboratory tests, interpret diagnostic data, track physiological monitoring systems, and conduct tomographic scans and noninvasive imaging procedures in nuclear medicine (Anderson & Jay, 1985; Hawkins, Day, Gustafson, Chewning & Bosworth, 1982; Kreps, Hubbard, & DeVita, 1987; Makris, 1983). *Medical informatics* improve health care delivery by increasing the sophistication of medical instruments, assisting research into epidemiology, and enhancing decision-making in clinical medicine. *Health informatics* increase the efficiency of health organizations by managing administrative (accounting, billing inventory, payroll), client care (admitting, appointment scheduling, dietary, laboratory, nurse scheduling, pharmacy), and general management control (budgeting, productivity analysis, utilization review) health information processing functions (Makris, 1983).

Computerization of medical records serves both clinical and administrative information functions in health care organizations by giving providers easy access to information for diagnosis and treatment and giving administrators records of health care services and resources. (The availability of computerized patient information also implies that health care organizations must be careful to protect the individual's information privacy.) Computerized appointment scheduling and shift scheduling has helped to solve many time-management problems in health care organizations (Nelson, 1981; Covvey & McAlister, 1980). Client history taking by computer has been used effectively to gather sensitive information anonymously, provide consumers with an interactive means of seeking health information, as well as to store and process client health information (Cohen, 1981).

Along with the many useful applications and benefits of computerized hospital information systems, several communication problems have also arisen. Some of the problems associated with the computerization of health care organizations include too much and too little access to health information (Brenner & Logan, 1980; Covell, Uman, & Manning, 1985; Kaplan, 1985). The storing of private medical records on computer files often allows people with questionable integrity who have no legitimate right to private medical information to access these data. For example, in 1986 information was leaked to the mass media from computer files of the Clinical Center of the National Institutes of Health (NIH) concerning the health care treatment being offered to Mr. Roy Cohn, an infamous New York lawyer. Mr. Cohn had repeatedly told media representatives that he was being treated for a liver ailment. Subsequent newspaper reports about his medical records from the NIH indicated he was being treated for AIDS, contradicting Mr. Cohn's previous statements and potentially causing him unnecessary distress. Other unwarranted uses of health information have occurred when suppliers of health care products and services have accessed computerized medical files to establish mailing lists for identifying potential customers. Problems concerning limited access to health information occur when those who need the information have difficulty getting it or understanding it, such as when the coding of information on computer files makes the data difficult to interpret or when data is omitted from the files.

There are many applications for computerized information storage and retrieval systems to help health care practitioners and consumers cope with the rapid expansion in health science literature and information that we discussed earlier in this chapter. Several different computerized health information systems have been developed to help users keep informed about relevant health care information. For example, "Medline is an on-line computer-based system to retrieve references to articles in biomedical journals. Toxline . . . is an information retrieval system for health professionals and scientists working in the areas of environmental pollution, occupational health and safety, poison control, pharmacology/toxicology, medicine, and related disciplines," and Avline is a computer-based retrieval system designed to help people recover stored information about health care related audiovisual materials (Harlem, 1977, p. 35-38).

Interactive computer systems are also useful in health care as diagnostic and educational tools. Computer programs have been designed that allow computers to interview health care clients about their general medical histories (Slack et al., 1966). Similar programs have been designed allowing computers to take psychiatric histories (Maultsby & Slack, 1971). Computers can provide diabetic individuals with dietary counseling and education (Slack et al., 1976). Hawkins et al. (1982) have developed an interactive computer program designed to adapt to the specific information needs of adolescent users in providing ". . . a number of health related topics such as smoking prevention and cessation, human sexuality, stress management, interpersonal relationships, alcohol and other drug abuse, diet and activity, and body image." Since this program protects the anonymity of its users and there is no human contact in giving or getting health information, the program provides a low-risk means for adolescents to acquire the specific health information in which they are interested. Computers offer the greatest potential of any media technology we have discussed in this chapter for providing health care professionals and consumers of health care with high quality health information. As more people have access to computers, computer technology will shift from being a primarily in-house use of interactive technology to being a public health education tool. The introduction of affordable, easy-to-use computer systems promises the eventual development of the computer as a mass media health communication tool.

Summary

Media technologies have provided important health communication tools that enable health care practitioners and their clients to reach beyond their personal ability to communicate to achieve their health care goals. The future development and growth of new media applications in health care promise to introduce exciting and innovative health communication tools and procedures. Media are extensions to our ability to communicate, and the complexities of modern health care demand all of our ingenuity in developing and utilizing powerful health communication media.

CHAPTER
7

Culture and Health Communication

Obi, a native of Africa, was studying geological engineering at a small college in the western United States. During his junior year, his father died. With a small inheritance and a collection of money from family members, his mother left Africa to be with her son in the United States.

Although she could not speak English, she was content to stay in the small apartment where she cooked, cleaned and was slowly introduced to the world of American technology while her son attended classes.

In the middle of the semester, Obi's junior engineering class was required to take a three-day wilderness field trip. He was hesitant to leave his mother since she could not communicate with anyone, but the field trip was required for course completion and his mother assured him she could manage.

The day after Obi left, his mother became ill. After several hours of agonizing pain, she managed to open the apartment door and stagger into the hallway. A next door neighbor found her shortly afterward and rushed her to the hospital. She was terrified and understood nothing, and she was mortified when strangers removed her clothes and started probing her body. She was of no assistance in indicating where her pain was located, and the emergency room doctor finally prescribed a tranquilizer. When the nurses tried to give her the medicine in pill form, she became agitated and would not take the medication. The doctor then prescribed an injection. She refused to lie still for this and she was held down while the shot was given. From that point onward, she huddled in a ball under the covers of her bed and the head nurse observed that the patient was as likely to die from fear as from her mysterious illness.

Obi's mother's condition worsened and exploratory surgery was scheduled. The physician was hesitant to proceed, however, until he had informed consent from the client or from her son. He tried to explain nonverbally what he was going to do to the patient, hoping he could secure her cooperation. She began moaning and screaming. This continued for four hours until the son finally reached the hospital.

As details were given to the son he was shocked. His mother had never been in a hospital and her beliefs were still firmly rooted in her African culture. Additionally, in her view she had been threatened by the nonverbal gestures of the physician as well as by the attempts of the nurse to hold her down while giving medication. Later, with the son's translation it was determined that the woman had appendicitis and that an operation was indicated.

What are the intercultural and ethical decisions that health providers should consider with a client such as this one? In this chapter we will focus on culture; in the next we will focus on ethics. At all times, we see these subjects as interrelated in health communication. Cultural and ethical behaviors — as well as interprofessional sensitivity — are prerequisites for effective health communication.

The case of Obi's mother reflects some of the many components of *ethnomedical systems* which are the culturally unique beliefs and knowledge about health and disease (Witte, 1991). Studying culture through ethnomedical models enables us to realize how culturally based beliefs about health and illness as well as wellness can affect a client's cure. Additionally, such study enables us to understand how western medical systems are focused on disease while naturalistic and personal systems focus on a holistic perspective.

Terminology

Just as different cultures sometimes have their own language, so does the language of intercultural communication. This section will define and explain some of the key words necessary to understand the material in this chapter. Borrowing heavily from the works of Samovar, Porter and Jain (1981) and the edited readings of Samovar and Porter (1991) we define *culture* as the deposit of knowledge, experiences, beliefs, values, attitudes, meanings, hierarchies, religion, timing, roles, spatial relations, concepts of the universe and material objects and possessions acquired by large groups of people in the course of generations through individual and group striving.

Intercultural communication, is the overall encompassing term that refers to communication between people from different cultural backgrounds. Often cross-cultural and transcultural communication are used synonymously (Samovar, Porter & Jain, 1981). These broadly used terms become confusing when it is not clear whether they refer to cultures within a country or between countries.

Interracial communication is the form of communication that occurs when the participants in the interaction are from different races. *Race* refers to a system by which humans are classified into subgroups according to specific physical and structural characteristics such as skin pigmentation, stature, or facial features. The three commonly recognized racial categories — Caucasoid, Mongoloid and Negroid — greatly overlap causing more similarities than differences (Henderson & Primeaux, 1981). For example, an interaction between a Japanese-American and an Iranian-American exemplifies interracial communication. On the other hand, a recently arrived Russian talking to the same Japanese-American exemplifies both interracial and intercultural communication. *Interethnic* refers to situations where the participants are of the same race but of different ethnic origins or backgrounds. *Ethnicity* refers to individuals who share a unique cultural and social heritage passed on from one generation another. A German-American talking to a Greek-American is an interaction involving members of different ethnic backgrounds whose members belong to the predominant North American culture and race. English-Canadians and French-Canadians also exemplify interethnic backgrounds since they are citizens of Canada but quite different in background, perspectives, viewpoints, goals and languages.

The term "Hispanic client" refers to ethnicity; the description "Black doctor" refers to race. In a society in which one in four people are people of color, none of us can afford to remain ignorant of the heritage and culture of any part of our population and therefore understanding both differences and similarities is important. *International communication*, on the other hand, refers primarily to communication between nations and governments.

A *subculture* is defined as a group of people with clearly identifiable values that exists within the geographical boundaries of a dominant culture. In the United States, for example, some of these subcultures are based on religious or regional definition, as well as on the definition of groups which deviate by choice from the national norms or culture. Kalish & Collier (1981, p.95) define the subculture of white middle-class males as follows:

> Among middle-class males of White or European ancestry will be found homosexuals, persons living on rural communes, militant advocates of Black supremacy, men who want to father children without marrying the mothers, men who wish to bake bread rather than buy it, men who refuse to eat meat, men who are in training to serve as guerilla fighters when the Communists take over the country and men who are addicted to heroin. The degree to which a culture will tolerate deviation and accept the conflicting values of subcultures depends on the values of the culture. Vegetarians are more tolerated than homosexuals; workers in communes are more tolerated than advocates of violence.

As the quote indicates, the complexity of studying cultures and subcultures is formidable but not impossible and it is a particularly important task when members of different cultures need to communicate to achieve mutual goals, such as the goals of health care.

While other definitions will be introduced throughout the chapter, these general terms will provide the background for much of the following discussion.

Culture

The word culture is often vaguely and unexplainably used. We talk about the "black culture" (with some groups, the term Afro-American is preferred), the "Asian culture" the "drug culture" or the "culture" of the community without clarifying the manner in which we use these terms. An understanding of culture is particularly important if effective communication is going to take place. In health care, for example, personnel must have an adequate perception of both their own culture and the culture of the client. Intervention can do more harm than good if the participants misinterpret behavior. This is evident in the case presented at the beginning of this chapter.

Culture provides humankind's most important assets — the ability to grasp the world and agree on what is real (Bauwens, 1978). "There is an inseparably close link between culture and communication. We cannot understand culture without reference to communication and communication without reference to culture" (Dissanayake, 1989, p. 105). Karl Deutsch (1966) concurs stating that culture is based on the community of communication which consists of social stereotypes including habits, language and thought which are carried on through various forms of social learning, particularly through methods of child rearing. One country can be host to many subcultures within its geographic boundaries. Within the United States, for example, women have a somewhat separate culture from men, blacks from Indians, and children from the elderly. In the area of health care, physicians have a culture difference from other health care providers. Language, friendship, eating habits, communication practices, music, social acts, economic and political activities, and technology dictate culture and its different groupings.

Often in the past, the importance of culture has gone unrecognized, particularly in regard to such areas as health care. However, a recent emphasis on the many facets of culture has stressed the importance of studying intercultural communication. Not only does the study of culture bring fresh insights into understanding the variability of human beings, but it aids us in solving communication problems between different groups. In the case of Obi's mother, the lack of understanding between well-meaning health providers and the client (an example of interracial and intercultural communication) prevented effective interaction from taking place.

Culture is intriguing, but it is also difficult to study and understand. Why someone eats certain foods, wears certain clothes, and uses certain language would be far easier to investigate if each person belonged to only one culture, but frequently cultures overlap. It is possible to be a sixty-year-old female American Indian physical therapist living in England. In such a case, many cultural influences interplay. Cultures are also difficult to perceive because we subconsciously absorb cultural constraints. Culture becomes a form of conditioning which is so subtle it cannot be isolated; it shows itself only through behavior which is a product of culture. For example, an American doctor or a nurse might be offended by a client who tried to stand too close to them, whereas in an Arab culture close proximity would be expected.

Discussions about culture often revolve around *cultural bias*. This refers to a tendency to interpret a word or action according to some culturally derived meaning assigned to it. The works of Edward T. Hall (1959, 1966, 1976) are particularly important in this regard. Hall discusses significant differences in how people of different countries and cultures use space, time, and context in culturally biased ways.

Time is seen as the exemplification of a culture's orientation toward the past, present and future. In many Western cultures we are time bound and quite dominated by concern with *monochromic* time (M-time). In an M-time culture, people value being on time and usually do one thing at a time. They are heavily management-oriented, and their appointments are heavily scheduled. M-time people are usually from highly developed Western cultures.

Persons in *polychronic time* (P-time.) are often from Mediterranean or South American cultures. They value doing many things at once and are often relationship oriented. Both kinds of times have their advantages. In health care, problems sometimes occur when people interact from different time perspectives.

Proxemics, or the use of space is also an important part of health communication. Space involves the distance between people as well as their physical orientation. Many persons from Arabic countries value close interaction where men often kiss each other; in European countries, the handshake is more than adequate. How a health provider organizes his or her office and how clients are placed in nursing homes are also examples of spatial issues.

Hall (1976) found a difference in how cultures utilize context. *Context* is the set of circumstances that surround situations. He determined that a *high-context culture* was one in which much of the information is exchanged in the physical context or internalized in the person. The American Indian culture and Asian cultures are high context where verbal skills are considered suspect and confidence is placed in nonverbal communication (p. 322). Alternatively, *low context cultures* have very explicit language codes and tend to prize verbal skills. The United States tends to be a low context culture along with Germany, Sweden and the Scandinavian countries. Understanding these contextual differences and presenting information to clients which stresses the verbal or nonverbal priority of their culture can reduce uncertainty and make health care more successful. The element of context permeates both written and spoken language, codes, patterns of organization and health care.

From the practical point of communicating effectively in a health care setting, one must decide how much time to invest in "contexting" the person with whom one interacts. For example, should a physical therapist explain the workings of the body, how physical therapy interacts politically with medicine, the workings of Medicare, and any number of issues with which he or she is familiar to the elderly client? Some clients might not be interested in this "contexting." However, their cooperation and effort might increase if they had a greater knowledge of physical therapy and all it could do for their welfare.

In studying intercultural communication, particularly in health care, it is particularly important *not* to focus entirely on traditional Western medical scientific models. Western and non-Western medical systems are social rather than logical and both are culturally determined. Non-Western systems sometimes emphasize homeopathic approaches which believe in returning the body to normalcy while Western systems tend to be allopathic or disease oriented. Bias toward one system or the other is often based on bias and acculturation rather than data (Payer, 1988). Stein (1990) warns us about the cultural prevalence of the traditional biomedical model which focuses on an allopathic medical model. He notes that the prevalent biomedical model stresses symptom removal and is largely authoritarian and cognitive rather than encompassing material that could be utilized from such areas as behavioral science.

Understanding cultural patterns other than time, space, and context are also important. As Purtilo (1978) illustrates, such issues as "bad breath" are quite often issues of cultural origin. Some cultures value garlic, others onions, and still others tobacco. Health professionals need to recognize many cultural factors as quickly as possible as they prepare to work with clients.

Acculturation Problems Between Subcultures

There is a cultural variance between members of any interaction when their perception of social objects and events as well as their use of the language is different because of their acculturation. *Acculturation* refers to the process of absorbing cultural traits.

An example of acculturation that is particularly significant to human beings is that of gender where the consequences of acculturation are very noticeable in most countries. Howard Stein (1990) contends that the health care system is designed around male values. For example, he argues that while the female value of "caring" is the ideal value for health providers, the nurturant values associated with care rank it far below the active, virile, masterful, and conquest virtues associated with the more masculine values of "curing." The gender biases that are associated with the biomedical culture are shown in Figure 7.1.

In addition to gender, there are many other factors, such as one's world view that affects the acculturation process.

World Views

A client's world view or view of society is important because these views also effect the perception of others. *World view*, for example, deals with one's attitude toward religion, the nature of humans, and of the universe. Attitudes about one's world view are subtle and do not reveal themselves easily. Our world view is so deeply imbedded in our psyches that we take it completely for granted and assume that everyone views the world as we do.

Figure 7.1   Masculine/Feminine Dualism in Biomedical Culture

Masculine Images and Values	Feminine Images and Values
Active	Passive
Doing	Being, becoming
Technological intervening, having a procedural orientation, prescribing medicine	Listening, talking
Control	Out of control
Cure, fix	Care, "hand-holding"
Doing to, manipulating, palpating, performing lab tests	Doing with another, touching
Physician, doctor	Therapist, counselor, nurse, social worker[a]
Biomedical science and technology	Social/behavioral science, social work
Science	Nature
"Hard science"	"Soft science"
Doctor	Patient
Individualism and "line of authority" or "chain of command"	Decision by consensus
Taking charge of situations	Waiting, "going with the flow," making decisions in a situational basis
Internal locus of control	External locus of control
Future time orientation	Past or present time orientation
Military, sports, business, and technology metaphors	Interactive metaphors, such as support, nurturance
Death as unnatural, but to be conquered	Death as natural, an inevitable part of life
Surgeon as epitomizing image	Psychiatrist, psychologist, family therapist, pastoral counselor[a]

[a] Although these professionals are viewed by higher status biomedical professionals as "feminine," members of these mental health or biopsychosocial specialties have in recent years been striving to divest themselves of the association with "feminine" values. Psychiatry has to a large degree attempted to disassociate itself from behavioral science and become more biologically oriented. Much psychotherapy has become focused on symptom removal and short-term effectiveness. The structural, strategic, and family-of-origin schools of family therapy (Salvador Minuchin, Jay Haley, and Murray Bowen, respectively) tend to be directive. As Nora Krantzler (1986) points out, American nurses are attempting to become associated with physicians' image of manipulators of technology (Stein, 1990).

Reprinted from *American Medicine As Culture*, Howard Stein, 1990, by permission of Westview Press, Boulder, Colorado.

Unwritten world views and belief systems are important to consider when dealing with matters of ethnicity and culture. American Indians view peyote as useful to physical and mental health; conservative Roman Catholics often believe in the value of pain and suffering. Third World cultures have developed kinship systems which have no legal ties but are important to a client's recovery. Within Hispanic communities the concept of machismo can cause men to ignore pain. Realizing these beliefs or checking them out with the patient or the family is vital to effective health care (Henderson & Primeaux, 1981).

In research directly related to intercultural communication, Collier (1988) found that while members of different cultures shared general communication rules, Mexican-Americans emphasized a relational climate, Black Americans stressed individuality in politeness and expression, and white Americans emphasized verbal ability. Additionally, Collier also found that for the most part, rules for conversation with members of one's own group were different from rules for intercultural conversations. If these differences exist within a country, it is easy to imagine how much more complex communication can become with people from other lands.

Bringing together world and ethnic views is particularly difficult for people living outside their country of origin. As Henderson and Primeaux (1981) note, black American culture is not African culture, nor is Mexican-American culture Mexican culture; the mainland Puerto Rican culture is not island Puerto Rican culture. Members of these cultures living in America are part of a *cultural amalgamation* — a synthesis of their own native and adopted American cultures. As members of different cultures improve their economic status, they often take on the characteristics of the majority culture and lose their ethnic identity.

All of these factors taken together make it important for the health care professional to realize that members of groups are not identical and that sensitivity is paramount in order to assist clients with their health care. The case study at the beginning of this chapter clearly illustrates how difficult it is to deliver effective health care when the client's world view and social orientations are not understood. We will focus on different health care models in four developed countries in the next section to illustrate issues health care providers may confront.

Medicine Across Four Cultures

One of the most innovative books written on the relationship between health, medicine, and culture in recent years is *Medicine and Culture* by Lynn Payer (1988). In this book, the well respected writer for the *New York*

Times gives some powerful examples of medicine and culture. Comparing four First World industrialized nations with similar mortality statistics, Payer found that all four internationally regarded health systems have quite different cultural views and treatments of different illnesses and diseases.

Each country was found to base its health care on national character and cultural norms. In France, the system seems to be based on Cartesian logic, and much of French medicine focuses on diseases of the liver and the stomach. The French discount statistics and studies; instead, they emphasize what they find "rational" or "reasonable" for the patient. In Germany, a country that stresses the heart, there is an authoritarian romantic model predominating with an emphasis on the blood pressure and the circulatory system. In England many doctors are kindly but paternalistic (their focus is on the stomach and the bowels!); in America, aggressive models based on viruses and germs predominate.

In researching treatments given in each of these countries for the same illness or disease, Payer (1988) found that one country's treatment of choice may be considered malpractice across the border. In general, treatment and diagnosis flow from how the particular culture views the body and its workings. In France where an emphasis is placed on beautiful, intact bodies, few hysterectomies and caesareans are undertaken by surgeons. In the United States, by contrast, these are some of the leading operations.

Payer's review of the cultural aspects of medicine in the United States focuses on the following aspects. American providers are aggressive and want to *do something*. American aggressiveness has mixed results. American physicians prescribe more diagnostic tests than are done in the other three countries. They prefer surgery to drugs. If drugs are used, they prefer higher dosages, particularly in the area of psychiatry. Surgery is more aggressive and is performed more often.

American clients are sometimes seen as suffering from nervous exhaustion and burnout as they battle the "enemy" — their disease. The client who is beating cancer is seen as the victor; while the person who succumbs is seen as a failure. Those who refuse treatment are seen as deviant.

In the United States, we are often condemned by health care providers in other nations for our inadequate treatment of chronic disease, for our hurry to find solutions without adequately evaluating the problem, and for sometimes having to repeat surgical or medical procedures.

The idea of the body as a machine is also seen as an American phenomenon. Payer relates the high rate of by-pass surgery (twenty-eight times that of some European countries) to the machine metaphor which contains a mechanical notion of the heart. Bruno Bettelheim, the recently-deceased child psychiatrist was critical of the machine approach noting this ignores the importance of assessing deeper issues. Anything that does not fit into the "machine" model is often denied not only quantification but even existence. As one doctor said in discussing childbearing centers, "We don't believe in taking an added risk in order to satisfy an emotional need. It's an indulgence" (Payer, 1988, p. 151).

On the positive side, technological innovations and research are most prominent in the United States. The "can-do" approach of medicine in the United States has been given credit for cutting the rate of heart attack and stroke. The American rate of heart attack has fallen by 40 percent in the last twenty years due to treatment, prevention, or both.

In contrast, other nations have many variations in philosophy regarding treatment. Germans use medication in smaller dosages. All of the other countries emphasize prevention to a greater extent than does the United States, and treatment for the chronically ill is given precedence.

Payer's conclusion is a powerful one which deserves reflection. She contends that choice of diagnosis and treatment is not necessarily scientific but based largely on cultural concerns. Health care providers and their clients need to be aware of the power of culture when they make health care decisions. They also need to reflect on the differing beliefs, values, attitudes, and world views that affect both their behavior and the behavior of the client.

Beliefs, Values, and Attitudes

The cultural impact of beliefs, values and attitudes strongly influence health care for both the practitioner and the client. Anthropology teaches us that disease, health, and illness are culturally defined. Beliefs, values, and attitudes express cultural codes and social circumstances as well as organic conditions (Stein, 1990, p. 21). *Beliefs* are basic units of thought establishing a relationship between at least two entities. They are ideas people hold about the truth or falseness of a given topic. Virtually any statement that begins with the phrase, "I believe that . . ." is a belief. Verbal beliefs are called opinions. *Values* are beliefs that evaluate or judge. They often involve good or bad or right or wrong statements.

Stein (1990) sees the *values* of current medicine as being control, activism, and doing as opposed to caring, conforming nondirective counseling, waiting, and doing nothing (p. 38). *Attitudes* are the cluster of beliefs relevant to some central object of judgment. For example, if I believe that cancer is contagious (a *belief*) I will think that it is bad to visit hospitals (a *value*) and my *attitude* toward visiting or being with anyone who has cancer will be negative. Attitudes are predispositions people have about whether to react positively or negatively to something. Beliefs are organized in a hierarchy that ranges from shared basic beliefs that seldom change to beliefs that are less rigid. However, beliefs and values that are central and rigid in one culture often change in another. What is more, values can change within a culture itself over different time frames. For example, in India a high cultural value was formerly placed on having large families. Now because of the need for population control in that country due in large part to a shortage of resources, values are changing. There is an increasing attitude on the part of government officials and individuals that smaller families are more desirable.

Attitudes have the components of cognition, effectiveness, and intensity or expectancy. These three elements interact to create the psychological state needed to react to objects and events in our environment. For example, if we believe that mental or physical pain should never be endured and we have no prejudices against pharmacological drugs, then our attitude system might be favorable to using pharmacological products such as Prozac and Demerol without much discrimination.

The importance of a client's beliefs, values and attitudes within his or her own cultural framework cannot be over-estimated. "A person's beliefs influence their perceptions of health and illness. Beliefs dictate which symptoms will be considered appropriate to take to a doctor, how patients will understand the cause and treatment of their illness, what patients expect of physicians, what personal and moral meanings patients will ascribe to their illness and how they will answer the perennial questions 'Why me? Why now? What did I do to deserve this?' Health care providers who ignore these beliefs overlook a powerful source of information and a potent tool for healing because evidence exists that knowing a patient's beliefs, values and attitudes can improve the outcome of the interaction" (Weston & Brown, 1989, p. 80).

Most interactions are medically centered, that is, they are based primarily on the beliefs of medicine. Mishler (1984) suggests an approach which focuses on the patient. This can be accomplished by such questions as, "What are you most concerned about? How does this illness disrupt your life? What do you think is happening to you?" Such questions begin to draw out cultural concerns as well as private client beliefs, values and attitudes. Additionally, they enable the health care practitioner to begin to understand the world view and social organization of the client as well as the other concepts presented in this chapter.

Social Organizations and Roles

In order to make sense out of this plethora of cultural considerations, members of a society establish social organizations which, in turn, designate roles for its members.

Social organization refers to the way a culture organizes its members and its institutions. Geography and roles are an important part of social organization. The institutions of society such as schools, churches, universities, armies, prisons, mass media, and the health care system convey the values of a certain culture.

Through unwritten as well as written codes of laws, values and stereotypes are conveyed by institutions. For example, the unwritten codes of health care in the United States have traditionally included a provision that physicians "always know best" and should have major control over areas in the realm of medicine. The courts are constantly being called in to decide if midwifery, homeopathic medicines, or herbal cures are violating the edict that only physicians can practice "medicine," a matter which is often a cultural as well as a legal determination.

Social organizations define the role each of us must play within the culture in such institutions as families, churches, and hospitals. In the past, these roles have been rigid and rather inflexible. The advantage of rigidity is that clear information about the role is conveyed. The disadvantage is that it is difficult to change roles as society changes.

Roles can stay the same across geographical boundaries, although cultural circumstances sometimes change the roles. For example, the fact that approximately 90 percent of Russian physicians are female would make the role of the physician different in Russia than in the United States. Health care professional organizations such as medical or nursing associations are prime arbitrators of professional socialization for the roles of their members. Not only do they govern who can or cannot belong to their organizations, they govern much of the unwritten code regarding the conduct of their members.

Roles of both the client and the health care provider are also influenced by the stigmas connected with particular health situations and by what we call the "religion of medicine." These subjects are discussed in the following section.

Stigma and Mystical Aspects of Health Care

Stigma, or loss of social identity and status, is a primary problem facing people seeking health care, and the stigma of an illness affects how roles are assigned in health care. *Stigma* is a social situation that occurs when a person's public image is "reduced in our minds from a whole and usual person to a tainted, discounted one" (Goffman, 1963, p. 3). Due to the perceived deviance associated with the sick role, those seeking health care often suffer from stigma. Media portrayals of health care consumers can reinforce the powerless stereotype embodied by the sick role (Cassata, Skill & Boadu, 1979). Cultural stereotypes often lead to stigma and to prejudicial treatment of many groups of health care consumers, such as AIDS sufferers (Hughey, Norton, Edgar, & Adamson, 1986), the aged (Kreps, 1986), the poor (Kosa & Zola, 1975), blacks (White, 1974), Hispanic-Americans, (Hoppe & Heller, 1975; Martiney, 1978; Quesada & Heller, 1977), women (Chesler, 1972; Corea, 1977; Mendelsohn, 1981), the mentally retarded (Baran, 1977), and the disabled (Braithwaite, 1985; Dahnke, 1982; Emry & Wiseman, 1985, 1981).

The cultural perspectives of the health care system by individual societies have a dramatic influence on health and health care. For example, Mendelsohn (1981) suggests modern American culture views health care as though it were a religion. The "religion of health care" is steeped in mysticism, too dark and mysterious for the average "parishioner" (patient) to understand. Consumers must have faith in the wisdom of the high priests and priestesses of health care (providers) to interpret the gospel of health care and direct health-preserving activities. Religion as a metaphor for health care reinforces the passive, almost obsequious, role many health care consumers adopt (Kreps & Thornton, 1984). The client's dependence on the mysticism and ritual of health care for controlling illness and providing care promotes unrealistic consumer expectations for health care outcomes. This places the provider in a one-up power position in the client/provider relationship, and discourages consumers from taking active roles in their own treatments (Ballard-Reisch, 1990; Becker, 1974a, 1974b; Blackwell, 1967; Colm, 1953; Crane, 1975; Gochman, 1969; Mechanic, 1972b; Myerhoff & Larson, 1976; Roth, 1957).

Divesting health care and stigma of their mystical hold on clients and providers is an important part of becoming a caring health care provider. Careful and effective communication combined with an understanding of one's own beliefs as well as the beliefs of others offer an excellent basis from which to proceed.

Reactions of the Individual to Cultural Bias

Up to this point, we have presented many factors influencing cultural communication and have discussed how a society organizes itself to deal with cultural concerns. The influence these cultural concerns have on the individual is our next topic.

A *personal cultural bias* is a tendency to interpret a word or action in terms of some assigned individual significance. Such personal bias can often result in prejudice. Most personal biases are also cultural, but because they occur at the unwritten or unconscious level, the individual is often unaware of his or her prejudiced views. An Indian health professional practicing in a community that is negatively biased toward Indians will lose some patients because of the community and personal interpretation of what "Indian" means. A Caucasian physician could conversely be disliked and mistrusted in an Indian community if bias against Caucasians is present.

Discrimination based on personal bias works craftily, evasively, and with stunning certainty. Both parties involved are inevitably injured by the interaction. In health care, where trust is such an important part of the relationship, misunderstanding through bias or prejudicial behavior can prevent healing at all levels (Purtilo, 1978, p. 126).

Personal biases greatly influence interaction, and the attempt to eliminate negative personal prejudices is an important part of maturity on the part of the health professional. Sidney Jourard (1964) spoke of the problems that could arise when a nurse allows those biases to affect care. His quotation also applies to all other health professionals who should substitute their profession as they read this quote.

> There are nurses who cannot care for patients who are known to be immoral. One of our students mentioned that with some young mothers of illegitimate children who were having their babies in a local hospital she, the nurse, would stay a minimum length of time and get out of the room as fast as she could. We can call this girl a "goodness specialist." There are white nurses who cannot care for Negro patients. Let us call these nurses "white specialists." There are nurses who are repelled by sex and who balk at taking care of patients who make passes. We might call these specialist "nurses of neuters."

> There are nurses who cannot take care of people whose behavior is at first bizarre and incomprehensible, as is sometimes true of so-called psychiatric patients. We might call these nurses "normality specialists." There are nurses who can do what is called for only with patients unconscious on the operating table. A conscious patient induces anxiety; threat, bashfulness, etc. We might call these nurses "coma specialists."

> There are nurses who can care only for Protestants. Catholics, Jews, Hindus, agnostics and Zen Buddhists arouse their anxiety and indignation and they provide only minimum care for people in these categories. We might call these nurses "Protestant specialists" (Jourard, 1964, pp. 135-136).

It is important to understand that personal biases are disseminated through *socialization*, the process by which members of a culture receive continuous, usually unanimous, reinforcement to behave in culturally approved ways. Socialization is conveyed through stereotyping, ethnocentrism and proselytizing. *Stereotyping* is the process that occurs when we, as individuals, convey our beliefs regarding such issues as equality, individuality, and social status and expect others to agree with us in some way. "Indians are always drunk," "Blacks are inferior," and "Blondes are dumb" are examples of painful and undocumented stereotypes perpetuated by some people. Vicious stereotyping in this century occurred when Adolf Hitler condemned the Jewish race as inferior and sought to eliminate it.

As can be seen, *stereotypes* are symbols intended to identify ethnic groups, races or subcultures. Generally, they are standard mental pictures used to oversimplify the characteristics of members of other groups.

Stereotyping is done because it makes communication easier. Through stereotyping we feel we know which groups we can feel more comfortable with and which groups are more likely to share our values. We develop stereotypes regarding status and roles, as well as ethnicity. For example, the physician as "godlike" is a stereotype (sometimes harmful to both physician and client), but it serves as a way to make the health care hierarchy clear to all parties.

Health care workers from other cultures are particularly disturbed by the stereotyping that locks members of their culture into simplistic groupings. One clinical worker was annoyed by the local residents' tendency to say "Haitian is like that, Hispanic is like that, you know those Italians are all alike . . ." She felt these stereotypes blinded people to the diversity within such groups (Brownlee, 1978, p. 23).

One of the major stereotypes in the United States regards aging. Consider the times you have heard the elderly referred to as old fogies, boring, garrulous, unproductive, and worthless. A harmful and untrue stereotype that combines ageism and sexism exists in the phrase "old ladies and tennis shoes."

Even though the elderly are the fastest growing population in the United States, this nation does not display respect or great concern for its gerontological population. The national bias in favor of youth is clear in the media, in entertainment, and in business. The stereotyping of our gerontological population will need to change in order for the country to meet the needs for services of this group as more people live longer.

As seventy-year-olds complete marathons, practice as physicians, and climb mountains, it is important to ponder why we have created myths which create the belief that only the young are superior in intellect, physical ability, sexual prowess and good looks.

Knowing that our stereotypes come from sensory inputs, it is important to become conscious of the negative views that are perpetuated in songs, movies, stageplays and comedy routines for all groups. While stereotypes will always exist, the well-educated, discerning individual will seek to understand the reason for their existence and will combat them when they are destructive.

Ethnocentrism, like stereotyping, is a major barrier to cultural understanding. It is the tendency to interpret or to judge all other groups, their environment, and their communication according to the categories and values of your own culture. Americans are seen as particularly ethnocentric by many groups. We are both benevolently ethnocentric (we judge others by our standards but still tolerate them) and militantly ethnocentric (we frequently force our values on others). Everett Klunjans, a Chancellor of the Honolulu East West Center once proposed that Americans should stop playing God and join the human race. He has indicated that he thinks it is time for Americans to develop a more humble style of relating to people. Ethnocentrism can be a serious problem in health care when the health practitioner is relating to someone from a different culture yet does not accept or respect the tenets of that culture. Getting impatient with a Hindu who won't eat meat or with an African who wears an amulet are examples of ethnocentric behavior (Sitaram & Cogdell, 1976).

Proselytizing is an attempt to force an intercultural perspective on others. It is the process of advocating that members of other culture groups adopt "your" view on religion, politics, government, or whatever else is at stake. Proselytizing takes place in health care when providers, or other clients for that matter, attempt to force their views regarding health or medicine on others. This is often done in an effort to get clients to "comply" rather than to cooperate.

The personal issues discussed in this section (bias, stereotyping, ethnocentrism and proselytizing) are difficult to overcome. Culture is perpetuated unconsciously and nonverbally. Awareness of bias, both personal and cultural, is the first step toward eliminating prejudices. Factors which can assist us in this process are presented in the next section of this chapter.

Factors Promoting Intercultural Interaction

There are many ways to improve intercultural interaction and address miscommunication caused by cultural factors. Historically most programs concerning health and health education have been designed for whites or are pre-existing programs adapted to an ethnic group by layering a thin veneer of cultural information over them. Tripp-Reimer and Afifi (1989) have developed models based on cultural assessment and negotiation that assist the providers in better understanding cultural issues.

Cultural assessment is the process of obtaining an overview of the characteristics of a client in order to identify needs. Topics in an initial interview include degree of affiliation with cultural groups, religion, patterns of decision making and preferred communication styles. The interviewer elicits cultural information that is problem specific. For example, if the client is seeking prenatal care, data is obtained about her feelings about being pregnant and the anticipated delivery and treatment as well as detailed cultural factors that influence intervention strategies. If the prenatal client needs help with exercise or diet, information would be collected on cultural patterns of eating and exercise.

After assessment, *cultural negotiation* or cultural brokerage takes place. Essentially, these negotiations are acts of translation in which messages, instructions, and belief systems are manipulated, linked, or processed between the professional and the client of diagnosis and preferred treatment. Several steps are followed:

1. Attention is given to eliciting the client's perception of the illness or problem.
2. Scientific information is provided with the acknowledgement that the client may hold different views.
3. If the client's perspective indicates that the behaviors suggested would be adaptive or neutral they are implemented; if not, negotiation continues until agreement on treatment is reached.

At no time during this assessment and negotiation process should the health care provider over-generalize or stereotype clients based on his or her cultural heritage. However, the provider should use cultural knowledge and background cues that will assist in providing the necessary health care assistance.

In establishing dialogue, the provider needs to identify the preferred communication style of the cultural group which includes use of the client's primary language when possible. Clients are seldom comfortable with first names. They need to be asked questions such as the following: "What do you want to be called? Is eye contact acceptable?" If communication appears to make the person uncomfortable, the assumption should be made that the problem is not always with the content but often with the process. It is most important not to be condescending or paternalistic. Translators are often desirable but when they are not available the provider should:

1. Speak slowly and make sure that the session lasts as long as necessary.
2. Make the sentence structure simple, but not simplistic.
3. Avoid technical terms (for example, use "heart" rather than "cardiac").
4. Do not assume the client understands but ask the client to explain and paraphrase.
5. Involve family and friends and a social support system.

In working with clients or health care personnel who are members of other cultures, there are other steps that can be taken to facilitate better communication. Most important, time must be taken to discover what kinds of special verbal or nonverbal information is necessary to establish effective interaction. What are the space needs of the individual from the other culture? Do they respond to touch? What kind of eye contact is considered appropriate to establish trust? Are there any special rules of protocol that should be followed? In the case study at the beginning of this chapter, an understanding and a focus on cultural differences would have provided more appropriate treatment for the mother from Africa.

One of the best ways to gather information about clients is to listen to their stories which can supply useful clues to their beliefs and values. While this may seem to be time consuming, in the long run it will actually save time and provide the information necessary to deliver a higher overall quality of care for the client. Time becomes important in the establishment of trusting relationships. The female proctologist and the male client from Mexico need to establish trust before an examination. The mainland Chinese female and the hurried American male gynecologist must do the same.

In conducting an interview with a person of another culture, it must also be remembered that the provider's cultural characteristics may influence the responses clients provide. Police stations and hospitals have recently begun to realize that rape victims respond better to a female and that women police officers and health providers should be utilized. Age, ethnicity, sex, educational level, and social class may greatly influence the information obtained in an interview.

One final caution! In establishing any new relationship with persons from another culture it is important to focus first on similarities. While differences are important, as we have already indicated in this chapter, similarities are also of value. A recent book on culture and communication quotes a Native American hospital administrator: "I feel you should start with a 'people' focus rather than a focus on differences. Similarities form a basis for relationships. Ask, 'What is common to human nature?' not 'What kind of pain does she have, a Navajo pain or an Anglo pain?'" (Brownlee, 1978).

A humorous story which reflects the necessity to listen carefully to persons of different cultural settings and to learn all you can about the person you are interviewing circulated on a college campus. The story tells of a researcher who spent thirteen years compiling a dictionary of one of Papua New Guinea's 700 tribal languages. She reported that her task wasn't easy. In fact, to assemble a list of verbs she had to act them out for the informant. For the word "jump" she jumped up and down in front of the village elder and recorded what he said. Six months later she found out that what he had said didn't mean "jump" at all. It meant, "Why are you acting so stupid?"

Interprofessional Relationships as an Intercultural Concern

> *When a frantic mother brought in a child who had just swallowed a coin, Sharon, a new radiology technician for a large group of physicians, took the x-rays and isolated the coin in the pictures. It presented potential harm as it was located near the trachea. The busy radiologist on call looked at the film quickly and, not seeing the coin, told the mother not to worry and to take the child home. Sharon was dismayed. Her initial interactions with the physician had been unpleasant ones, and she was told when she was hired that she should not interfere or express opinions in front of clients or families. What should she do?*

Up to this point, this chapter has been devoted to a discussion of the intercultural characteristics that can greatly affect the health care practitioner-client relationship. In this section of the chapter we will emphasize the culturally related professional constraints that affect the interprofessional relationships between health care providers. Often caused by different acculturation, these constraints (often stereotypes) are:

1. *Different educational backgrounds.* Physicians generally receive more initial formal training than do other health professionals. Nurses receive more applied training. Perceptions from these different kinds of training models often collide.

2. *Different career patterns.* Physicians are often self-employed while many others are employed by institutions. Even in the institutional settings, physicians are often not beholden to the organizational structure.

3. *Jargon and semantic differences.* Different words have different meanings to different professionals. For example, when physicians describe a nurse as "cooperative," they mean that the nurse obeys orders. When a nurse talks about a "cooperative" physician, he or she means that the physician is treating them equally.

4. *Class differences.* Many physicians make more money, travel with different groups of people, have more prestige, and interact more often with those higher in authority. Additionally, they generally have more authority in the health care system.

5. *Gender and racial differences.* Most physicians are white middle class males even in the 1990s. The lower the status of the health care professional, the more likely the role will be filled by a woman or minority. Not only is there a difference in status but also a difference in pay. While over 70 percent of health care workers are female, most high paying status positions in the health care field are staffed by males.

Difficult patterns of communication that often develop between nurses and physicians are often blamed on male-female cultural differences. In a study of nurses, the words nurse and feminine were linked by the subjects representing different cultures. The words "nurse" and "feminine" were perceived as good but weak — stereotypes limiting nurses' abilities to deliver health care (Austin, Champion & Tzeng, 1985).

6. *Value and focuses.* While the physician sees his or her functions as curative, nurses and other health providers see their function as caring. Admitting officers see their function as being efficient, as do administrators. These conflicting goals or functions can cause confusion and conflict, for both the client and the health provider or administrator.

7. *Professional isolation.* Largely due to the factors listed above as well as to time constraints, professionals are often isolated from each other. Without frequent informal as well as formal contact, differences and misunderstandings between members of the various professions grow and become divisive. Tensions that build as professionals work together can be traced to different bureaucratic and professional goals, as well as to divided loyalties — and once again to culture. The hospital administrator has to be loyal to the hospital board while at the same time responding to staff and client needs. The nurse has to be concerned about peer relationships, relationships with physicians, and the care of the individual client. Additionally, tensions are caused when every individual working in health care settings brings his or her prejudices and stereotypes to the work setting. The doctor who does not respect females will have difficulty with female nurses; the respiratory therapist who does not like Hispanics will have difficulty responding to orders from a Hispanic physician.

In attempting to solve interprofessional problems, the solutions are very similar to the solutions given for intercultural communication. For example, spending time and listening to others is of paramount importance. Professionals need to learn problem-solving techniques which enable the parties involved to look at mutual problem areas and apply techniques designed to improve the decision-making process, the major focus of the interprofessional interaction. The example regarding the radiology technician at the beginning of the section exemplifies a type of constraint that can be caused by different acculturations. Health care providers must generate procedures that enable them to work together for the client's welfare. Such procedures need to reinforce the value of all those participating in the health care system. An ethical perspective, discussed in the following chapter, is also very important in interprofessional relationships.

Summary

In this chapter, the influence of culture on our lives has been examined, emphasizing the belief that an understanding of culture is important for effective communication in health care. A look at culture often explains the reasons for lack of communication between the sexes, the ages, and the races. An understanding of culture explains our use of time, space, and context. Being aware of culturally related terminology, as well as differing beliefs, values and attitudes is a requirement for any health care professional. Having an enriched understanding of world views, social organization roles, stigma, and cultural differences among practitioners enables health care workers to better serve their clients.

Individuals and organizations are often unconsciously biased and need to devote resources to uncovering and correcting biases, stereotyping, ethnocentricism, and proselytizing that sometimes contribute to ineffective or inadequate care. An awareness that our system of medicine is different and not always better than those of other nations is also important.

It is also important to acknowledge that health providers within the same country often misunderstand each other's professional culture and context, a situation compounded when each party to the interaction is originally from a different country or culture.

Cultural assessment and negotiation techniques can help professionals deal with cultural issues. An awareness of the cultural implications of interprofessional relationships can also improve the health care climate.

CHAPTER
8

Ethical Communication in Health Care

Susie was a hospitalized twelve-year-old girl diagnosed with terminal cancer. Her parents asked the physician not to tell her she was dying, and the physician had written those orders on the chart. Late one evening, Susie asked the duty nurse, to whom she had become attached, if she was going to live. What are the ethical obligations of the nurse?

The beliefs, values and attitudes of an individual, a family, or a social group greatly influence ethical decisions. In this chapter, we will focus on the relationship of communication to ethical decision making in health care. In addition to discussing this relationship, the chapter will discuss relevant ethical theories and principles and focus on methods for taking ethical action.

At all times, the relevance of culture to ethics and communication will be stressed. Our underlying premise is that the beliefs, values, and attitudes that individuals and groups hold influence their ethical decisions and are determined by their culture.

Ethics in Health Care

Decisions regarding health care that involve moral issues are called *bioethical decisions*, and the field of study of these life-involving moral decisions is called bioethics. The term "bioethics" literally means the ethics of life. It is the critical examination of the moral dimensions of decision making in health related contexts and in contexts involving the biological sciences.

Matters such as deciding where resources including money and time should be allocated in health care have moral dimensions. For example, policy makers must decide whether prenatal care or by-pass operations should receive Medicaid funds when there is not enough money for both procedures.

The process of moral decision making as well as the transmission of these decisions into actual behavior is of relevance to the health communicator since the relationship of communication to ethics cannot be overemphasized. Often the health professional has the ideals and values necessary to be ethical but does not know how to translate his or her beliefs into ethical action. When values collide, as they often do between members of a team or between health care providers and clients or families, communication strategies such as conflict management are important. Ethics without communication becomes meaningless. Communication is the channel through which ethics are established and conveyed.

In the past, bioethics has primarily been studied from a philosophical viewpoint; the codes of the various health professions are based on these philosophical theories. Any reader interested in reviewing these theories is encouraged to do so through the perusal of texts on bioethics. In this chapter, we will focus primarily on the relationship of bioethics to communication.

For example, the case utilized at the beginning of the chapter demonstrates many communication related bioethical issues such as *informed consent, paternalism, interpersonal responsibilities* in health care, as well as the issue of *children's rights*. Cultural matters are important variables in these issues. For example, how a culture views its youth, parental control, and the relationship between nurses and physicians concern both ethics and culture.

Whether young children, like twelve-year-old Susie (the terminally ill child discussed in the beginning of this chapter), are capable of making their own decisions or of absorbing the truth is one of the major issues in biomedical ethics today. Certainly it poses an interesting dilemma for those concerned about children's rights. In this case, the nurse did tell Susie she was seriously ill and was almost fired for volunteering that small amount of information. The assumption was that only the physician could or should release that data. In addition to who should tell, the Susie case raised the question of how much or what to tell a client. This is a dilemma of *informed consent*, defined as the knowing consent of an individual or his or her legally authorized representative. A highly respected national report on this topic emphasizes the following communication related issues:

1. While informed consent has substantiation in law, it is essentially an ethical imperative.
2. Ethically valid consent is a process of shared decision making based upon mutual respect and participation. It is not just ritual.
3. Informed consent is important for people of all cultures. It should be required for *all* practitioners in their relationships with *all* clients. It is not a luxury for a few well-educated or well-informed individuals.
4. Health care providers should not ordinarily withhold unpleasant information simply because it is unpleasant. Most reports on informed consent find that members of the public do not wish to have bad news withheld from them.
5. Shared decision making based on mutual respect is ultimately the responsibility of individual health care professionals and not systems which fragment responsibility.
6. Clients should have access to the information they need to help them understand their conditions and make treatment decisions.
7. Techniques such as having clients express, either orally or in writing or both, their understanding of the treatments should be explored.
8. Educators should prepare physicians and nurses to carry out the obligation of informed consent.
9. Family members should be involved in informed consent when the client chooses to involve them in the process or when they need to represent the interests of clients unable to communicate their own needs.
10. While decision making between the consumer and the health provider is the ideal, groups organized for such processes, such as ethics committees, should be utilized when appropriate. They can express a continuum of views on moral issues.

11. Limits must be placed on the range of acceptable decisions that advocates or guardians can make beyond those that apply when a person makes his or her own decisions. (President's Commission, 1982).

While these are ideal generalizations, they are difficult to carry out. Clients who are incompetent need the special guidance of advocates acting in their behalf. It is not easy to determine the "moment of competency or capability" for children such as Susie or for the very ill.

Did the nurse who told Susie that she was seriously ill exceed her responsibility and violate the nurse-physician-parent relationship, or was she acting as a very moral advocate when she truthfully answered her client's question? Communication becomes an important part of bioethical decision making as these rights and responsibilities are negotiated.

The current focus on bioethics and its concerns are probably greater than at any other time in history. A surge in medical technology plus a concern about the ethical aspects of health care account, in part, for this trend. Abortion and birth control, for instance, are heavily contested issues in the United States, and the rhetoric surrounding them is vociferous. In abortion and other ethical debates, communication techniques can at least help clarify the issues when values collide. For example, debate on abortion or allocation of resources can be conducted under fair guidelines, where beliefs, values, and attitudes can be sorted out. An example of such communication occurs in the household of Dan and Sidney Callahan, both respected writers in the fields of morality and ethics. They hold diametrically opposed positions on the issue of abortion. Yet they have worked and lived together for over thirty-eight years.

In addition to communication techniques, it is also important to understand the ethical principles involved with a particular issue. *Confidentiality* requires that a person's right to privacy be balanced with the safety or health of others. Abortion requires the balancing of the rights of autonomy and privacy with potential rights of the fetus and of society. The right to life and the right to death involve justice, respect for life, and caring and concern for others. An understanding of the principles each culture holds dear is an important part of the decision-making process.

Legal and Professional Codes and Oaths

Many persons in health care consider themselves *professionals*. This term usually refers to a group of people who are educated according to certain guidelines, have a special vocabulary or jargon, and are given special privileges, including the privilege of policing their own profession. In return they have the responsibility to deliver high-quality care to their clients. It is assumed that the professional is committed to a higher goal than his or her self-interest and that the final and most important dimension of the professional responsibility is a moral one (Camenisch, 1983).

Critics of the professions, such as Illich, et al. (1977), see the professions as dangerous to health care consumers. Believing that professions are organized for economic advantage rather than consumer protection, they suggest less professionalization of "experts" and the development of more control and expertise by consumers. Their criticisms have been supported by others, particularly feminists who argue that women, in particular, need to take more control over their own bodies, especially in the area of reproduction.

In order to assist professionals in their ethical responsibilities, and to hold professions accountable, the professions have developed codes and oaths. Historically these codes and oaths have been designed to focus on values and ideals as well as to protect the professional from the infringement of others.

One of the authors of this book assigned prehealth professional students to find the code of ethics that pertained to their professions. Attempts to find these codes in local libraries or to obtain them from professionals in the community were time consuming and largely unsuccessful, indicating the lack of actual emphasis placed on the codes by professionals and others.

Critics of these codes indicate that most codes are much too general and lack definitional terms. Most do not prioritize the values they discuss nor do they effectively address the fundamental issue of what is best for the client rather than what is best for the profession. While these codes are important in that they focus on moral principles and duties, it is clear that much more than a code is needed to ensure ethical behavior and that current codes and oaths are not adequately enforceable.

Some recent studies of ethics and the professions encourage professionals to investigate their codes and play a role in rewriting and enforcing these documents so they will focus more on what is good for the client rather than the profession (Camenisch, 1983). Additionally, professional conferences and meetings are encouraged to include sessions on ethical issues.

The Social Issues of Death, Dying, and Aging

As life expectancy increases, an aging population will suffer more from chronic illness and sometimes lingering death. Additionally, technological advances can keep persons "alive" on highly sophisticated equipment for an indefinite time, making a natural death an infrequent occurrence. Some of the ethical issues involved with death concern autonomy and paternalism, as well as the quality versus the sanctity of life. Addressing these dilemmas involves communicating about issues that are emotionally loaded, such as euthanasia. Active listening, self-disclosure, as well as a discussion of feelings emotions, and family history are important. As Kreps (1988) suggests, effective communication about death and its associated feelings provides therapeutic effects to allow individuals to cope with the multiple issues that death entails.

Policy makers and health providers are encouraging persons to discuss and record their wishes regarding dying and cessation of treatment through advanced directives, such as living wills and durable powers of attorney. In order to do this, persons will need to discuss their wishes with family and friends.

A Plan for Ethical Action

In the past, clinicians and others making bioethical decisions have been advised to utilize traditional approaches and theories such as the prioritization of principles, vices, or virtues.

However isolating principles and virtues is not enough if ethical action does not take place, and it is our contention that without action, ethical thought is meaningless. That is, a physician who believes in truth telling but who does not tell the truth in day-to-day practice is not *being* ethical.

In the remainder of this chapter, we present a stair-step model for ethical action called the ESSAA method which incorporates traditional decision-making elements as well as guidelines for implementation and evaluation. *ESSAA* stands for ethical readiness, sorting, solving, acting and assessing. While this method focuses on ethical decision making, it can also be applied in general to the decision-making process. An outline of this stair-step process is presented in Figure 8.1. We will discuss the elements of this scheme in the following pages.

Step One: Educating for Ethics

In order to prepare for moral decision making, decision makers must have at least an elementary understanding of bioethics. The role of education in this area is subject to debate. One side argues that moral patterns are determined in childhood, and education is not helpful. Proponents of education argue that moral development can take place throughout the lifespan. Recently there has been an emergence of programs and projects

Figure 8.1 ESSAA Method of Ethical Decision Making

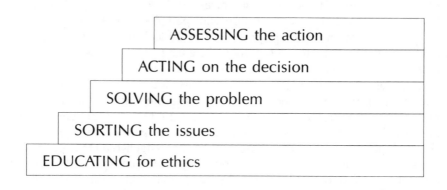

designed to sensitize as well as to educate people from school children to adults about values and morality.

Conservatives argue that values are best taught in the home; those who disagree argue that many families are not capable of accomplishing this task. Lawrence Kohlberg (1981) of Harvard, now deceased, was one of the leaders of the current movement to teach values education. Proponents of Kohlberg's methods continue to test many school based programs.

Recently, some philosophers have stressed the importance of character education, which is education based on virtues such as courage and integrity. At the same time, Gilligan (1982), Nodding (1984), Ruddick (1989) and others have focused on caring as the basis for ethical decision making. While these writers do not discount principles or virtues, they suggest that a general attitude of caring and an emphasis on the relationships involved in the ethical decision are equally important. Such relationship oriented perspectives focus on effective communication as pivotal in expressing these relationships as part of the bioethical decision-making process.

Colleges, organizations, and professional schools often promote values education. Courses in universities or colleges, week-long seminars, and even educational events over the weekend are examples of the many ways health professionals can educate themselves about the ethical dilemmas in health care today.

Part of the preparation process also includes deciding who are the appropriate decision makers in regard to the particular ethical decisions. As indicated in the chapter on groups in health care, ethics committees have increasingly become involved in advisory decisions regarding moral issues in health care. Ethics committees do not make decisions; instead, they assist others. The general rule is that they don't become involved in cases unless asked to do so by one of the appropriate parties, such as the physician or nurse. However, most ethical decisions are made by individual health care providers in conjunction with patients and families.

Once a situation calls for some kind of ethical decision making, it is important to recognize the importance of creating an atmosphere conducive to thoughtful reflection. The institution or setting in which the ethical dilemma is taking place should emphasize the importance of ethical behavior and encourage personnel to act accordingly (Levine-Ariff & Groh, 1990). However, most bureaucracies are not geared to these concerns, and individuals will need to create their own safety zone for behaving ethically. For example, if an ethics committee is asked to establish a DNR policy for a hospital, members need to know they will be given a time and place for consultation and discussion and that any policy they develop will be supported by the medical staff, the nursing staff, and the administration if it is to be implemented.

Part of the preparation process for ethical action involves awareness of the cultural factors that are part of the ethical decision, particularly those that are unconscious or nonverbal. In the last chapter, we discussed bias, prejudice, and the background for different beliefs, values and attitudes as well as world views. Being aware of our own belief system and the manner in which that system influences decision making is particularly important. If you believe that women cannot make good decisions about reproduction, you obviously have some gender bias. If you think that the particularly high rates of heart disease and breast cancer among black people are caused by the fact that they are careless about their health, you have vestiges of racial bias. If you are a nurse who thinks that all doctors are insensitive and thoughtless, you have professional bias. In any of these cases, you are incapable of putting yourself in what John Rawls (1971) calls the original position where you try to make decisions from an objective, unbiased point of view.

In summary, the education stage for effective decision making consists of achieving an ethics background, developing an atmosphere in which effective decisions can be made, identifying the relevant decision makers, and becoming aware of cultural factors such as bias and prejudice that may affect decision making.

Step Two: Sorting the Issues

Stage two of ethical decision making involves the categorizing and sorting of issues. Certainly, in making ethical decisions and taking ethical action, it is important to know how participants to the dilemma perceive the fact, value, and policy issues. Determining their point of view means listening to their stories. *Narrative theory* is the nomenclature given to listening and evaluating stories, and it is appropriate methodology for this stage of bioethical decision making. Examples of the narrative approach can be found in the works of Howard Brody (1988), Arthur Kleinman (1988), Warren Reich (1987), and Barbara Sharf (1991).

The contribution of narrative theory to the behavioral science is becoming more apparent in the last few years. Fisher (1987) argues that human beings are by nature story tellers, and it is by listening to these stories that we can understand the topics, history, or issues that are important to an individual or group. The increasing use of stories to illustrate moral issues (Reich, 1987) or medical interviews (Sharf, 1991) demonstrates the effectiveness of a narrative approach to health care ethics.

In addition to listening it is important to pay attention to feelings and emotions in decision making. The moral issues of health care arouse intense emotions in the provider as well as the consumer of health care. In the past, providers were told to hide or to disguise those emotions; mental health professionals today suggest the opposite. Such feelings as empathy need to be displayed by both parties to the health care interaction. Additionally, it is valid to have negative emotions, and these need to be identified and dealt with by those concerned. Rationality and emotion need to be balanced for effective decision making to take place.

When decision makers in health care or other areas do not listen to the stories of involved participants, unforeseen and sometimes disastrous consequences can result.

> *Several years ago in California, a young girl was diagnosed with leukemia. Her parents were afraid of the consequences of the suggested medical treatment which included surgery, radiation, and chemotherapy. Shortly after they moved to Nevada, however, their daughter was taken from the school playground and placed in a foster home without parental consent. They were charged with neglect. The California authorities had notified Nevada social services who, without any discussion with the parents decided that the child's best interests could only be protected in a foster home where traditional medical treatment could be authorized and undertaken.*

> *The case was taken to court where the judge ruled that the parents, not social services nor the medical profession, had the authority to make decisions regarding their daughter's welfare. The child was returned to her parents who tried desperately to save her through alternative methods of cancer treatment such as laetrile. These*

methods were futile, however, and she died. It is quite possible that she would have been saved by conventional treatment if the participants to the decision would have listened to each other's stories.

As this case made its way through the court and the newspapers it became clear that none of the participants had understood or listened to each other. The parents were afraid of traditional treatment. They were not given the opportunity to meet other parents and children who had successfully completed treatment. The physician, though well-meaning, had been abrupt with explanations of the treatment he was suggesting and distrustful of the parents' ability to make a good decision regarding their daughter's health care. The social services personnel were especially uninformed. Without any conversation with the California physician, the parents, or Karen herself, social services disrupted a family by taking their daughter from them and failing to respect their rights to make their own health care decisions (Melton, 1984),

Both this case and the Susie case presented at the beginning of the chapter demonstrate complex ethical dilemmas affecting children, but they are also cases which raise issues that are pertinent at any phase of life development. It is only through listening to others that we can obtain the information necessary to make good qualitative decisions for all phases of the life span.

In addition to listening to others as we sort the issues and to becoming aware of the place of feelings and emotions in ethical decision making, we need to be aware of how theories, the law, principles, and stereotypes affect our decision making. Traditional ethics has dealt with ethical issues primarily through a reliance on theories such as deontology and utilitarianism. Utilitarians generally believe that actions should be taken on behalf of the greater good of the individual and society. Deontologists believe that duty or principle should be the major focus. Sometimes these theories collide and they are not seen as particularly helpful in day-to-day clinical practice. For example, in the above case, a utilitarian might have argued that the greater good for the individual and society would have been to force traditional treatment on the child against the parents' will. The deontologist might have argued that the principle of autonomy should receive the highest consideration. Since there is merit in both positions, it is sometimes difficult to see how decision making based on theory can be helpful even though a knowledge of these theories is incumbent on anyone studying ethics. Alternative ethical theories can be reviewed in a bioethics textbook.

Knowledge of the law is also important but not a prerequisite for ethical understanding. It is important to remember that ethical and legal considerations are not always compatible. For example, the law in South Africa has, until recently, supported a system of apartheid which many people view as an unethical system. "Law aims to secure and defend an established order, a status quo. Ethics speaks to human potential and development, to ever higher ideal of service, human betterment and self-realization" (White, 1990). Individuals or groups preparing to examine ethics need to sort out these distinctions.

In sorting the issues, it is also important to emphasize that the ethical principles involved are sometimes different for the individual and the societal group involved with the decision. The issues of AIDS is illustrative. It is clearly in the interest of the person with the HIV infection to have the principles of confidentiality and autonomy respected. It is easier to obtain or retain jobs and insurance if no one knows a person has AIDS. The interests of the person with AIDS, however, do not always coincide with the interest of society. For example, preserving the confidentiality of the person with AIDS might work to the detriment of persons who might share needles or have sexual contact with that person. Balancing the needs of the individual and society to provide justice is an important part of ethical decision making. In recent years there has been greater emphasis on considering the influences of individual freedom and autonomy in conjunction with the common good.

Stereotypes, discussed in chapter 7, often affect ethical decision making. For example, because the elderly client is often stereotyped as being incompetent, informed consent is not always requested or required, and there is often a tendency to view the elderly as incapable of making their own decisions. The following example illustrates how a cultural stereotype against the elderly affects ethical decision making:

> *Mr. Edwards, age 66, had a pre-existing heart condition and was admitted to the hospital after a serious accident in which his wife was killed. Although his larynx was paralyzed, he could write on a chalkboard.*
>
> *He indicated that he had a living will which provided that he not be kept alive by any heroic measures in the event of any serious heart condition. The physician, however, noted on the chart that the man's son had left orders that all possible action should be taken when necessary. On the day the man's second heart attack occurred, he was resuscitated. The staff felt that because he was "elderly," the son should make the decision. There was no evidence that the client was incapable.*

In this case, ethicists would see paternalism as a real issue since the client's wishes were not followed. *Paternalism* refers to an action that is seen as advocating a person's interest but which in reality limits the person's behavior, desires, or freedom of choice.

Truth telling is a vitally important ethical issue involving communication. Sissela Bok (1974), a leading contemporary ethicist and expert on truth telling, indicates that the truth is important in most societal situations, including health related ones. An analysis of truth telling by the health communication expert can clarify truth telling issues and make the health care professional aware that there are many communication related variables. The level of trust between professional and client is important to truth telling as is self-disclosure. Additionally, diplomacy or its lack can also affect the way the client receives the facts about his or her illness. It is our suggestion that sometimes difficult truth telling situations should be role played with colleagues or others so that the right words can be used in the actual situation. Many of us who believe in the truth have a difficult time telling it!

One of the most serious day-to-day ethical issues for health care professionals involves confidentiality and privacy. Computers, large bureaucratic settings with multiple records, and the many health professionals involved in a client's care are all factors that conspire to invade an individual's privacy or right to confidentiality.

It is a general moral rule that health professionals should not violate a client's confidentiality except when necessary to preserve the life or health of someone else. In day-to-day reality, however, the client's privacy is violated. Many hospitals have computers in which client records can be seen by anyone. Doctors, nurses, and other professionals in the health care setting often become hurried and careless with client information.

Solutions to this problem are complex and depend in great part upon an individual health care provider's ethical discretion. Not letting curiosity get out of bounds when a health care professional is not involved with the actual case and being aware of the importance of privacy for the client's physical and mental well-being are two important considerations.

Advocacy is another ethical issue that involves either assisting or defending the client. An advocate supports either action or non-action, and often the advocacy view of health care providers collides with other alternatives. For example, nurses are sometimes uneasy about their role in strongly encouraging clients to sign informed consents. Yet physicians can threaten to report them for refusal to follow orders if they don't obtain the informed consent, thus making it difficult for them to act as advocates for their client/patient. Nevertheless, most bioethicists would agree that even in difficult situations, advocating (through action or nonaction) on a client's behalf is a prime ethical duty of health professionals based on the principle of beneficence, which is doing good.

Common to these ethical issues is the importance of clear and accurate communication. All the good will and philosophical intention to be ethical becomes meaningless if communication is misconstrued. It is the argument of the authors of this book that health care professionals cannot act ethically if they do not practice competent and strategic communication. Taking time to listen and to make sure the client understands instructions, medications, or the implications of treatment is of paramount importance. Conveying factual information without frightening clients or family is an equally important part of ethical behavior. Learning not to overstate a case is also a skill which can contribute to the conveyance of rights and responsibilities. We do not argue that being ethical or communicating accurately are easy skills to learn or maintain, but we do argue that learning and maintaining them is an important part of being an ethical health care practitioner.

The communication expert is helpful in ethical discussions when he or she can utilize knowledge of group dynamics and interpersonal skills to sort out such concerns as theoretical considerations, the limitations of the law, and the conflicts between the individual and the community, as well as other communication and ethical principles involved.

Step Three: Solving the Problem

After the issues are examined, it is important to gather as many solutions as possible in resolving ethical dilemmas. One of the most successful strategies for decision making is brainstorming, which was discussed in chapter 4. Utilizing this method, creative solutions can be maximized. Groups using the brainstorming technique effectively must follow the rules: all suggestions are permissible, judgement should be avoided during the idea generation phase, and ideas should build on each other.

Many decisions initially seem to pose only two alternatives; the brainstorming process will often provide several possibilities. This process focuses on communication or processual techniques that can assist in solving ethical dilemmas.

Identifying alternative solutions to a complex decision is one step; evaluating those alternatives is another. Prioritizing the alternatives is much easier once an individual or group has spent adequate time analyzing the problem and its possible consequences. The answer to the dilemma needs to be workable. Ethical, economic, and political consequences need to be recognized if the ethical decision is to be turned into action. If you are not realistic about the constraints of institutions and political systems, action in many instances, will not take place.

When serious ethical matters are at stake, and the institution is not ready to consider them, some people turn to *whistleblowing* — the process by which an individual or group finds it necessary to share information outside the normal reporting channels. Whistleblowing should be a last resort for matters of conscience because this process often results in negative consequences for the whistleblowers, their families, and others. While whistleblowing can be very courageous, it is seldom easy. Often it can be avoided if people with similar interests band together and advocate change within the institutional setting utilizing diplomacy, public opinion, and group strategizing. If these methods don't work, and a client's or colleague's welfare is at stake, then the individuals need to consider careful ways to inform others while seeking support for their own actions (Thornton, 1988). Whistleblowing is an important communication activity.

Even with all these techniques at hand, solving problems is not always possible:

> *Ida Jones is an 63-year-old woman who survived a stroke and is in a nursing home. Although she signed a living will, she is being forced to live with a hydration and nutrition tube that she does not want, because the nursing home has a regulation that will not allow the removal of tubes. Since it is the only reputable nursing home in the small town in which she resides, her family hesitates to move her. At this point her family feels that there are no potentially workable solutions, but they are hoping to eventually change the nursing home policy. Others in her small town are beginning to talk about the necessity for an ethics committee which will serve nursing homes in the area for consultation on issues such as this. Solving ethical problems such as this one is seldom easy, and ethics sometimes takes time and patience.*

Step Four: Acting Ethically

One of us consulted with the new ethics committee of a well-run and well-respected hospital a few years ago. The committee, one of the first in the state, was excited about its tasks and set about the process of educating its members regarding ethical issues of health care. They hired consultants in several areas and became well-educated regarding the issues. However, when a hospital physician brought them their first case for consultation, they were unable to have their decision implemented!

Ethics without action is meaningless. In order for action to take place, the ethical decision you or others make must be shared with the appropriate parties. Once again, communication is vital. Parties involved need to know the reasons for the decision and what needs to be done to implement it. The old phrase, "timing is everything" is useful here, particularly when the decision is controversial or life threatening. It is important to act in a timely manner and keep key people informed.

It is also crucial to notify people in power at the time decisions are implemented. For example, if a hospital ethics committee recommends the withdrawal of the respirator from the brain-dead victim of brutal wife abuse and the physician agrees (thus causing the victim's prominent husband to be charged with murder), the hospital administrator and the public relations staff need to be notified. Even though they are not part of the ethical decision-making process, they can torpedo ethical action if they are not included.

Sometimes, in the implementation process of a decision, the facts change or the decision is found to be inappropriate. There is nothing wrong with going back to the conference table to discuss other alternatives. Many decisions in health care *are* reversible.

Step Five: Assessing the Decision

Once a decision has been made and implemented and time for reflection has taken place, it is important to bring the decision makers back together for assessment. In a supportive atmosphere, participants need to review the ramifications of the decision to utilize this information for the future. Reflection is appropriate to examine how future decisions of the same kind should be assessed. Would you make the decision again in the same way? Were the appropriate people involved? Was the process of implementation appropriate?

Sometimes decisions lead to policy changes. Do you need more cases of the same kind before that policy making takes place? Do laws need to be changed? You need to learn from your successes as well as your mistakes.

Lastly, it is sometimes important that decisions be evaluated and reevaluated at different times, especially if the facts change or if the results and ramifications were not the expected ones. Ethical decision making that incorporates all these steps: educating, sorting, solving, acting and assessing usually results in thoughtful ethical implementation.

Summary

This chapter applied concepts from communication and culture to the ethical issues of health care, asserting that communication is the channel through which ethics is established and conveyed.

Traditional ways of studying ethics by reflecting on principles and theories were briefly reviewed and a method of bioethical decision-making was introduced. Throughout the chapter, the importance of translating ethical talk into ethical action was stressed.

CHAPTER 9

Communication and Health Promotion

Gail and her husband Sam were eager to bring their newborn baby daughter, Patricia, home with them from the hospital. Although Gail had only been in the hospital for two days, they were more than ready to leave the hospital and get on with their lives. They had been very apprehensive about the childbirth process, especially about going through labor and delivery; but the whole event progressed just like they had been told it would. It was amazing to them how much they had learned from the weekly childbirth classes they had attended for the past few months and how helpful the exercises they learned in class were. Even though Gail experienced quite a bit of pain and discomfort during labor, with Sam's coaching she was able to concentrate on performing the breathing exercises they had practiced in class to work through the labor and delivery pains and experience *a relatively trouble-free natural childbirth. Sam provided her with a lot of support and encouragement during the birthing process, and Gail was glad he was there to help and share the experience with her.*

Baby Patricia was a strong and healthy infant and needed only a day or so in the hospital's well-baby nursery before she could be discharged from the hospital. The obstetrics ward nurses brought baby Patricia to Gail's hospital room and taught her how to breast-feed the baby, and before long the infant was nursing vigorously. The nurses instructed Gail and Sam about the safest ways to bathe and care for Patricia to keep the baby healthy once they took her home. The hospital also provided them with a new-baby gift basket full of infant care literature, baby supplies, and infant formula to bring home with them. Sam brought their new infant car seat with him to the hospital on the day of Gail and Patricia's discharge. He knew, from what he had learned at the childbirth class, how important it was to use an infant car seat for safety. He was especially glad he brought it when the hospital staff insisted on verifying that an approved car seat was available for Patricia before they would discharge her to her parents. Sam drove home carefully, while Patricia slept peacefully in her car seat, and he and Gail dreamed about what the future held in store for their young family.

Health Education and Health Promotion

This case clearly illustrates the role of communication in health promotion. Gail and Sam were provided with a great deal of relevant health information and personal support to help them prepare for a successful childbirth and to help them care for baby Patricia. The childbirth classes taught them about the labor and delivery process. It helped them develop and practice strategies for relieving the pains of labor and delivery. It also helped to prepare them for their roles as parents by teaching them how to maintain their child's health. The obstetrics ward nurses also engaged in health promotion activities when they taught Gail how to nurse and care for her new child. The hospital engaged in health promotion when they required the use of an infant car seat, as well as when they provided Gail and Sam with infant care supplies. The relevant health information the childbirth class, the obstetrics ward nurses, and the hospital provided to Gail and Sam reinforced the importance of their parental role as the primary health care providers for their child and will help promote the baby's health and the health of the whole family.

In chapter 6 we described health education as the process by which health information is disseminated to specific audiences. Communication is the primary force that fuels health education because communication, whether interpersonal communication or mass-mediated communication, is the process by which *relevant health information* is conveyed to those audiences. Relevant and persuasive health information provides individuals with both rationale and direction for adopting health-promoting behaviors. *Health promotion* is an important outcome of the use of strategic communication in health education efforts, where individuals who acquire relevant health information use this information to take charge of their own health and make enlightened health care choices. Yet, the communication process by which health information is disseminated is deceivingly complex. "Health information dissemination efforts must be strategic and adaptive to effectively reach and influence the health beliefs, attitudes, and behaviors of desired audiences. The unique cultural, educational, and linguistic attributes of different audiences must be taken into account when creating and communicating health messages intended to reduce health risks and encourage health preserving behaviors" (Kreps & Atkin, 1991, p. 648). In this final chapter, we will examine the role of communication in health promotion, summarize many key issues presented in earlier chapters, and identify strategies for communicating to promote public health.

Communication and Health Promotion Campaigns

In 1985, the National Heart, Lung, and Blood Institute (NHLBI) established a National Cholesterol Education Program based on the recommendation made at a consensus conference of experts held a year earlier by the National Institutes of Health (NIH) about how to lower cholesterol levels to reduce the risk of heart disease (McGrath, 1991). Epidemiological research suggested that a large percentage of American adults were at risk for heart disease because of high blood cholesterol levels. A 1983 survey suggested that while many Americans recognized the importance of lowering cholesterol levels to reduce the risk of heart disease, only about a third of all Americans had their cholesterol level checked and only about 3 percent actually knew their cholesterol level. The primary goal of the campaign was to encourage adults who had not had their cholesterol levels checked to do so. The initial message of the campaign was "know your cholesterol number" (McGrath, 1991, p. 661).

Public service announcements were developed for television, radio, magazines, and newspapers to encourage the general public to have their cholesterol levels checked and to know their cholesterol numbers. "Message testing indicated that the messages should (a) emphasize that high blood cholesterol could affect anyone and has no symptom, (b) appeal to people's curiosity about the existence of a number that expresses their blood cholesterol level, (c) convey the idea that something can be done about high blood cholesterol, and (d) reinforce people's identification with healthy, fit individuals" (McGrath, 1991, p. 661). Evaluation data collected in 1988 indicated the education program, along with other public messages about cholesterol, had raised the public's awareness and altered behaviors regarding the campaign goals. The number of Americans having their cholesterol levels checked increasing from 35 percent before the campaign was introduced to 59 percent, and the percentage of Americans who actually knew their cholesterol levels increased from 3 percent to 17 percent (McGrath, 1991).

This case history clearly illustrates the value of health communication campaigns in influencing health behaviors and promoting public health. Please recognize, however, that a great deal of planning and strategy went into developing and implementing this health education program. Formative research was conducted to help the campaign planners understand the current status of public health beliefs and behaviors regarding blood cholesterol and heart disease. Epidemiological research clearly established the relevance of the goals of the campaign; strategic message design and channel selection was used in developing and implementing the communication campaign, and summative evaluation research was used to evaluate the influences of the campaign on public health behaviors. The effectiveness of health communication campaigns are dependent upon careful planning and strategy in program development, implementation, and evaluation (Kreps & Maibach, 1991; Rogers & Storey, 1987).

Health Promotion and Health Risk Prevention

A primary goal of health promotion is to help people identify and avoid serious health risks and, when necessary, to help them seek appropriate health care treatment. Modern science has identified many factors that increase the risks different groups of people have for contracting life-threatening health problems such as cancer, heart disease, and AIDS (Relman, 1982; Rosen, 1976). Health promotion experts often develop strategic health communication programs and campaigns to educate the public about a wide range of serious health threats and to encourage adoption of healthy behaviors (Rubinson & Alles, 1984; Tones, 1986). Public health can be promoted by the development and implementation of health communication programs that help the public recognize serious health risks and that persuade the public to adopt strategies avoid these risks.

Many different health promotion campaigns have been implemented over the last decade or so to provide consumers with risk prevention information concerning such issues as: resisting drug abuse (Flay, 1986); encouraging good nutrition (Kaufman, 1980; Levy & Stokes, 1987); preventing heart disease, (Flora, Maccoby & Farquhar, 1989); discouraging drunk driving (Atkin, Garramone & Anderson, 1986); promoting smoking cessation (Bauman, Brown, Bryan, Fisher, Padgett & Sweeney, 1989; Flay, 1987); and encouraging safe sexual practices (Edgar, Hammond & Freimuth, 1988; Brown, 1991). These campaigns were designed to help audiences that were at high risk for encountering each of these specific health problems to resist and avoid these serious health risks. Health communication is a crucial element in this preventive approach to public health care because the provision of relevant and persuasive health information is a primary social process that empowers people to take charge of their lives by directing health preserving activities (Kreps & Maibach, 1991; Reardon, 1988).

Health communication campaigns are generally designed to help the public recognize health risks, promote self-management of health, gain access to state-of-the-art prevention and treatment techniques, and implement appropriate strategies for minimizing health risks (Atkin, 1981; O'Donnell & Ainsworth, 1984). Health communication campaigns often employ a wide range of message design strategies and use many different channels of communication (such as interpersonal counseling, support groups, lectures, workshops, newspaper and magazine articles, billboards, radio/television programs and public service announcements, as well as computer based information systems) to disseminate relevant health information to targeted publics. In recent years, modern campaigns have often integrated interpersonal, group, organizational, and mediated communication to effectively disseminate health information to specific at-risk populations (Atkin & Wallack, 1990; Reardon & Rogers, 1988). To the extent that such health communication efforts are successful, they can lead to the prevention of health risks. But, to be effective, health promotion campaign planners must use the most appropriate channels of communication and message strategies to help relevant publics recognize, evaluate, and respond to specific health constraints (Kreps & Maibach, 1991).

The development of effective health promotion communication campaigns is very complex. Health promotion planners cannot assume that mere exposure to relevant health information will lead directly to desired behavior changes (Edgar, Hammond & Freimuth, 1989; Portnoy, Anderson & Eriksen, 1989; Tones, 1986). There is a tenuous and multifaceted relationship between communication and long-term behavior change that must be addressed. Campaign planners must take into consideration the nature of the health risk, the specific audience targeted, and the health behaviors to be influenced when making difficult decisions about the best message strategies and communication channels for reaching and influencing targeted audiences (Flay & Burton, 1990; Rogers & Storey, 1987). Campaign planners must realize that exposure to campaign messages may lead to audience awareness only when messages are heeded; audience awareness may lead to changes in knowledge only when campaign messages are comprehended; changes in audience knowledge may lead to changes in beliefs only if the arguments made in the messages are accepted; and even then, changes in audience beliefs might or might not lead to changes in attitudes, intentions, and ultimately behaviors (Flay, Di'Tecco & Schlegel, 1980).

Communication Campaigns and Social Marketing

Modern health promotion efforts have increasingly adopted a *social marketing* approach to communication campaigns, where health behavior innovations are viewed as products to be sold to consumers (Lefebvre & Flora, 1988; Solomon, 1989; Wallack, 1990). By viewing health promotion as a marketing issue, campaign planners recognize that mere exposure to health risk prevention messages may not be enough to make a "sale." Rather, they must develop specific persuasive communication strategies to sell health innovations to specific target audiences. There are four major principles of social marketing, often referred to as the "Four P's" (Products, Prices, Placement, and Promotion) that are used to guide the development of persuasive communication campaign strategies. According to these principles, social marketers should:

1. Create a product that will appeal to a specific target audience.
2. Establish a price (according to economic, psychological, or social costs to consumers) for the product that will be attractive to the target audience by minimizing perceived costs and providing incentives for "buying" the health innovation.
3. Identify ways to place the product, through the strategic use of communication channels, to get the target audience's attention.
4. Develop marketing messages to promote the product to show audiences how to adopt the health innovation.

Audience Analysis

Sophisticated health promotion efforts carefully examine the audience to be targeted. To be effective, a campaign must clearly reflect its target audience's concerns (Kotler, 1975). Recall our discussion of audience analysis in chapter 6, as well as our discussion of communication and culture in chapter 7. To develop strategic health communication messages, the messages must be matched to the key cultural attributes of the audience for whom they are intended. Health promotion communication campaigns must appeal to the specific audience targeted since audience members who do not perceive the campaign as personally relevant are unlikely to pay attention to, interpret, recall, or heed the advice offered in health promotion campaign messages (Ajzen & Fishbein, 1980; Kreps & Maibach, 1991; Bandura, 1986; Petty & Cacioppo, 1981).

Audience analysis is used to identify target audience members' attitudes, interests, and understanding of campaign topics, helping campaign planners predict audience reactions to campaign messages (Dervin, 1989). Audience analysis provides campaign planners with information about consumers' involvement, knowledge, experience, and values concerning campaign issues and goals, as well as about the many cultural factors that may influence audience members' responses to campaign messages (Bandura, 1986; Grunig, 1989).

Health promotion campaigns generally segment (subdivide) large diverse audiences into smaller and more homogenous target audiences so the campaign can be directed to a group composed of members with similar attitudes and health orientations (Kotler & Roberto; 1989). *Audience segmentation* can be directed according to geographic factors (the location of the target audience), demographic factors (identifying characteristics of members of the target audiences), behavioral factors (the target audiences' involvement with the campaign topic), and organizational factors (the organizational networks of which target audiences are a part), or even by a combination of these different factors (Kreps & Maibach, 1991). A recent successful campaign to control tobacco use illustrates the use of an organizational segmentation strategy. The target of this health promotion campaign went beyond the individual smoker to focus on influencing organizations by encouraging health systems, planning commissions, industries, businesses, and schools to develop and implement local smoking control ordinances and work site smoking control policies (U.S. Department of Health and Human Services, 1989).

Design Issues

Effective health promotion efforts begin with clear, specific, and realistic campaign objectives, since campaign objectives are used to direct the campaign. In sophisticated health promotion efforts, research and theory are used to guide campaign activities to help achieve campaign objectives. *Formative research*, conducted to help guide and refine the campaign, is conducted to collect data about concept and message development for creating and selecting effective messages for specific audience (Atkin & Freimuth, 1989). *Process evaluation research* is used to assess the progress of campaign activities in achieving campaign objectives. *Outcome evaluation research* is used to determine the impact and cost-effectiveness of a campaign as well as why the campaign did or did not result in specific outcomes (Kreps & Maibach, 1991).

Communication theories can help campaign planners predict, explain, and prescribe strategies for addressing health risks at individual, interpersonal, group, organizational, and societal levels of analysis (Bandura, 1986; Kreps & Maibach, 1991; McQuire, 1989; O'Hair, Kreps, & Frey, 1990). For example, *diffusion of innovation theory* (Rogers, 1983; Rogers & Kinkaid, 1981), which suggests that important members of social networks (opinion leaders) strongly influence the innovation adoption behavior of other network members, can be used in health promotion campaigns by encouraging opinion leaders to deliver campaign messages to target audience members. Simoni, Vargas, & Casillas (1982) did successfully use diffusion of innovation theory in just this way when they trained shamen (medicine men) to disseminate relevant health information to rural Mexican villagers as part of a health promotion campaign.

Communication Channel Issues

Health promotion campaigns are dependent upon the selection and use of the best channels for communicating strategic messages about relevant health information to the public. Campaign planners must determine which communication channels (such as film, television, radio, computers, print media, or interpersonal communication) will most effectively accomplish their campaign objectives. Three communication characteristics are often used to select the best channels for campaigns: 1) *reach*, how large an audience can be communicated with via the channel; 2) *specify*, which particular groups or individuals can be communicated with via the channel; and 3) *rate of influence*, how credible is this channel of communication with those individuals it reaches (Kreps & Maibach, 1991). Interpersonal channels, for example, are often described as having low reach, high specificity, and a high potential rate of influence, while mediated channels are generally characterized by higher reach, lower specificity, and lower potential rates of influence (Kreps & Maibach, 1991). Many health promotion campaigns utilize multiple channels of communication to maximize the strengths of individual channels, while minimizing any channel limitations (Flay & Burton, 1990; Rogers & Storey, 1987).

Conclusion

This book has examined the important role of communication in promoting public health. The interrelationships between communication, health information, and health promotion have been touched on in each of the book's chapters. The key functions that interpersonal, group, organizational, and societal communication perform in providing health information to the public have been described. We have stressed the importance of partnership and cooperation between health care providers and consumers in health care, as well as interprofessional cooperation and coordination between interdependent health care providers. We strongly advocate:

1. The development of human communication competencies by health care providers and consumers;
2. The evaluation of moral issues and use of ethical communication strategies in health care;
3. The development of interpersonal empathy, as well as the use of therapeutic communication in health care relationships;
4. The humanization of communication policies and procedures in what is too often an over-bureaucratic health care system;
5. The development of sensitivity to and respect for cultural differences between participants in the health care system;
6. The strategic dissemination of relevant health information through all appropriate communication channels (from interpersonal to mass mediated) to educate health care providers and consumers, as well as to empower the public to resist health risks and make responsible choices about health and health care.

Bibliography

Aguilera, D. (1967). Relationship between physical contact and verbal interaction between nurses and patients. *Journal of Psychiatric Nursing*, 11, 13-17.

Ajzen, I., and Fishbein, M. (1980). *Understanding attitudes and predicting social behavior*. Englewood Cliffs, NJ: Prentice-Hall.

Albrecht, T., and Adelman, M. (1987a). *Communicating social support*. Newbury Park, CA: Sage.

Albrecht, T., and Adelman, M. (1987b). Communicating social support: A theoretical perspective. In T. Albrecht and M. Adelman, *Communicating social support* (pp. 18-39). Newbury Park, CA: Sage.

Alpert, J. (1964). Broken appointments. *Pediatrics*, 34, 127-32.

Arndt, C., and Laeger, E. (1970). Role strain in a diversified role set parts I and II. *Nursing Research*, 19, 253-259, 495-501.

Arntson, P. (1985). Future research in health communication. *Journal of Applied Communication Research*, 13, 118-130.

Arntson, P., and Droge, D. (1987). Social support in self-help groups: The role of communication in enabling perceptions of control. In T. Albrecht and M. Adelman, *Communicating social support* (pp. 148-171). Newbury Park, CA: Sage.

Atkin, C. (1981). Mass media information campaign effectiveness. In R. Rice and W. Paisley (eds.), *Public communication campaigns*. Beverly Hills, CA: Sage.

Atkin, C., and Freimuth, V. (1989). Formative evaluation research in campaign design. In R. Rice and C. Atkin (eds.), *Public communication campaigns*, 2nd edition (pp. 131-150). Newbury Park, CA: Sage.

Atkin, C., Garramone, G., and Anderson, R. (1986, May). *Formative evaluation research in health campaign planning: The case of drunk driving prevention*. Paper presented to the International Communication Association conference, Chicago.

Atkin, C., and Wallack, L. (eds.). (1990). *Mass communication and public health: Complexities and conflicts*. Newbury Park, CA: Sage.

Atman, N. (1972). Understanding your patient's emotional response. *Journal of Practical Nursing*, 22, 22-25.

Austin, J. K., Champion, V. L., and Tzeng, O. C. S. (1985). Cross cultural comparison on nursing image. *International Journal of Nursing Studies*, 22, 231-239.

Ballard-Reisch, D. (1990). A model of participative decision making for physician-patient interaction. *Health Communication*, 2, 91-104.

Bandler, R., and Grinder, J. (1975). *The structure of magic I: A book about language and therapy*. Palo Alto, CA: Science and Behavior Books.

Bandura, A. (1986). *Social foundations of thought and action: A social cognitive approach*. Englewood Cliffs, NJ: Prentice-Hall.

Baran, S. (1977). TV programming and attitudes toward mental retardation. *Journalism Quarterly*, 54, 140-142.

Barnett, K. (1972). A theoretical construct of the concept of touch as it relates to nursing. *Nursing Research*, 21, 102-110.

Barnlund, D. (1976). The mystification of meaning: Doctor-patient encounters. *Journal of Medical Education*, 51, 716-725.

Barnlund, D. (1968). Therapeutic communication. In D. Barnlund (ed.), *Interpersonal communication* (pp. 613-645). Boston: Houghton-Mifflin.

Basch, C. E. (1987). Focus group interviews: An underutilized research technique for proving theory and practice in health education. *Health Education Quarterly*, 219, 359-366.

Bates, E., and Moore, B. (1975). Stress in hospital personnel. *The Medical Journal of Australia*, 2, 765-767.

Bauman, K. E., Brown, J. D., Bryan, E. S., Fisher, L. A., Padgett, C. A., and Sweeney, J. (1989). Three mass media campaigns to prevent adolescent cigarette smoking. *Preventive Medicine*, 17, 510-530.

Bauwens, E. (1978). *The anthropology of health*. St. Louis, MO: C.V. Mosby Company.

Bayley, C. (1986, October). *Growing an ethics committee*. Paper presented at the Ethics Committee Revolution: Coming to Terms with Substance and Process conference, Rancho Mirage, CA.

Becker, M. (1974a). The health belief model and personal health behavior: Introduction. *Health Education Monographs*, 2, 326-327.

Becker, M. (1974b). The health belief model and sick role behavior. *Health Education Monographs*, 2, 409-419.

Beckhard, R. (1972). Organizational issues in the team delivery of comprehensive health care. *Milbank Memorial Fund Quarterly*, 50, 287-316.

Bellah, R., Madsen, R., Sullivan, W., Swidler, A., and Tipton, S. (1985). *Habits of the heart*. New York: Harper and Row.

Benjamin, A. (1981). *The helping interview*, 3rd edition. Boston: Houghton Mifflin.

Bennis, W., and Nanus, B. (1985). *Leaders: The strategies for taking charge*. New York: Harper and Row.

Bennis, W. (1989). *Why leaders can't lead*. San Francisco: Jossey-Bass.

Benson, H. (1975). *The relaxation response*. New York: Avon Books.

Bernier, C., and Yerkey, A. (1979). *Cogent communication: Overcoming information overload*. Westport, CT: Greenwood Press.

Bettinghaus, E. P. (1988). Using the mass media in smoking prevention and cessation programs: An introduction to five studies. *Preventive Medicine*, 17, 503-509.

Blackwell, B. (1973). Patient compliance. *New England Journal of Medicine*, 289, 249-252.

Bok, S. (1974). The ethics of giving placebos. *Scientific American*, 231, 17-23.

Booth, R. (1983). Power: A negative or positive force in relationships? *Nursing Administration Quarterly*, 7:4, 10-20.

Bostrom, R. (1970). Patterns of communicative interaction in small groups. *Communication Monographs*, 37, 257-263.

Boyer, L., Lee, D., and Kirschner, C. (1977). A student-run course in interprofessional relations. *Journal of Medical Education*, 52, 183-189.

Braithwaite, D. (1985, November). *Impression management and redefinition of self by persons with disabilities*. Paper presented to the Speech Communication Association conference, Denver.

Braverman, B. (1990). Eliciting assessment data from the patient who is difficult to interview. *Nursing Clinics of North America*, 25, 743-750.

Brenner, D., and Logan, R. (1980). Some considerations in the diffusion of medical technologies: Medical information systems. In D. Nimmo (ed.), *Communication Yearbook 4*. New Brunswick, NJ: Transaction, 609-23.

Brownlee, A. (1978). *Community, culture, and care: A cross-cultural guide for health workers*. St. Louis: C.V. Mosby Company.

Brownlee, A. (1978). *Community, culture, and care: A cross-cultural guide for health workers*. St. Louis: C.V. Mosby Company.

Brody, H. (1988). *Stories of sickness*. New Haven, CT: Yale University Press.

Brown, J. D. and Einsiedel, E. F. (1990). Public health campaigns: Mass media strategies. In E. B. Ray and L. Donohew, *Communication and health: Systems and applications* (pp. 153-170). Hillsdale, NJ: Erlbaum.

Brown, M. H. (1990). Defining stories in organizations: Characteristics and functions. In J. Anderson (ed.), *Communication Yearbook 13* (pp. 162-190). Newbury Park, CA: Sage.

Brown, W. J. (1991). An AIDS prevention campaign: Effects on attitudes, beliefs, and communication behavior. *American Behavioral Scientist*, 34, pp. 666-678.

Brownlee, A. (1978). Community, culture, and care: A cross-cultural guide for health workers. St. Louis: C. V. Mosby.

Burge, S. (1981). Audiovisuals. In C. Reuss and D. Silvis (eds.), *Inside organizational communication* (pp. 169-186). New York: Longman.

Burke, R., Weir, T., and Duncan, G. (1976). Informal helping relationships in work organizations. *Academy of Management Journal*, 19, 370-377.

Burns, J. M. (1978). *Leadership*. New York: Harper and Row.

Calder, B. J. (1977). Focus groups and the nature of qualitative marketing research. *Journal of Marketing Research*, 14, 353-364.

Callahan, D. (1990). *What kind of life?* New York: Simon and Schuster.

Calnan, J. and Barabas, A. (1972). *Speaking at medical meetings*. London: William Heinemann Medical Books.

Camenisch, P. (1983). *Grounding professional ethics in a pluralistic society*. New York: Haven Publications.

Caron, H. (1968). Patient's cooperation with a medical regimen. *Journal of the American Medical Association*, 203, 922-926.

Carroll, J., and Monroe, J. (1980). Teaching clinical interviewing in the health professions: A review of empirical research. *Evaluation and the Health Professions*, 3, 21-45.

Caserta, J. (1989). The loss of self. *Home Health Care Nurse*, 7, 5.

Cassata, D. (1983). Physician interviewing and counseling training. *International Journal of Advanced Counseling*, 5, 297-305.

Cassata, D., and Clements, P. (1978). Teaching communication skills through videotape feedback: A rural health program. *Biosciences Communications*, 4, 39-50.

Cassata, M., Skill, T., and Boadu, S. (1979). In sickness and in health. *Journal of Communication*, 29, 73-80.

Cassell, E. (1985). *Talking with patients: Volume 2 Clinical technique*. Cambridge, MA: MIT Press.

Cassella, C. (1977). *Training exercises to improve interpersonal relations in health care organizations*. Greenvale, NY: Panel Publishers.

Charney, E. (1983). Patient-doctor communication: Implications for the clinician. *Pediatric Clinics of North America*, 19, 263-279.

Chenail, R. (1991). *Medical discourse and systematic frames of reference*. Norwood, NJ: Ablex.

Chenail, R., Douthit, P., Gale, J., Stromberg, J., Morris, G., Park, J., Sridaromont, S., and Schmer, V. (1990). It's probably nothing serious, but . . .: Parents' interpretations of referral to pediatric cardiologists. *Health Communication*, 2, 165-187.

Chesler, P. (1972). *Women and madness*. New York: Avon Books.

Cline, R. W. (1990). Small group communication and health care. In E. Berlin Ray and L. Donohew (eds.), *Communication and health: Systems and applications* (pp. 69-91). Hillsdale, NJ: Erlbaum.

Cline, R. W. (1983). Interpersonal communication skills for enhancing physician-patient relationships. *Maryland State Medical Journal*, 32, 272-278.

Cline, R. W., and Freeman, K. (1988, May). *Asking the right questions: A qualitative analysis of AIDS in the minds of heterosexual college students*. Paper presented to the International Communication Association conference, New Orleans, LA.

Cohen, C. (1988). Ethics committees. *Hastings Center Report*, 18, 11-20.

Cohen, M. (1975). Medication error reports. *Hospital Pharmacy*, 10, 166.

Cohen, S. (1981). Experience with a computerized medical history system in private practice. *Proceedings of 5th Annual Symposium on Computer Applications in Medical Care*. Silver Springs, MD: IEEE, 121-123.

Cohen, S., and Syme, S. L. (eds.). (1985). *Social support and health*. Orlando, FL: Academic Press.

Collier, M. J. (1988). A comparison of conversations among and between domestic culture groups. How intra and intercultural comparisons vary. *Communication Quarterly*, 36, 122-144.

Colm, H. (1953). Healing as participation: comments based on Paul Tillich's existential philosophy. *Psychiatry*, 16, 99-111.

Corah, J. L., O'Shea, R., and Ayer, W. (1985). Dentist's management of patients' fear and anxiety. *Journal of the American Dental Association*, 110, 734-736.

Corea, G. (1977). *The hidden malpractice: How American medicine treats women as patients and professionals*. New York: William Morrow.

Cousins, N. (1979). *Anatomy of an illness as perceived by the patient*. New York: Norton.

Covvey, D., and McAlister, N. (1980). *Computers in the practice of medicine*. Menlo Park, CA: Addison-Wesley.

Cowen, E., Gestin, E., Boike, M., Norton, P., Wilson, A., and DeStefano, M. (1979). Hairdressers as caregivers I: A descriptive profile of interpersonal help-giving involvements. *American Journal of Community Psychology*, 7, 633-648.

Cowen, E., McKim, B., and Weissberg, R. (1981). Bartenders as informal interpersonal help agents. *American Journal of Community Psychology*, 9, 715-729.

Crane, D. (1975). The social potential of the patient: An alternative to the sick role. *Journal of Communication*, 25, 131-139.

Cranford, R., and Dodera, A. E. (1984). *Institutional ethics committees and health care decision making*. Ann Arbor, MI: Health Administration Press.

Dahnke, G. (1982). Communication between handicapped and non-handicapped persons: Toward a deductive theory. In M. Burgoon (ed.), *Communication Yearbook 6* (pp. 92-135). Newbury Park, CA: Sage.

Dangott, L., Thornton, B., and Page, P. (1978). Communication and pain. *Journal of Communication*, 28, 1-6.

Davis, M. S. (1968). Variations in patients' compliance with doctor's advice: An empirical analysis of patterns of communication. *American Journal of Public Health*, 58, 274-288.

Davis, M. S. (1971). Variations in patients' compliance with doctor's orders: Medical practice and doctor patient interaction. *Psychiatric Medicine*, 2, 31-54.

Davis, M., and Eichorn, R. (1963). Compliance with medical regimens: A panel study. *Journal of Health and Human Behavior*, 4, 240-249.

Day, F. (1973). The patient's perception of touch. In E. Anderson, et al. (eds.), *Current concepts in clinical nursing* (pp. 266-275). St. Louis: Mosby.

Day, S. (1975). *Communication of scientific information*. New York: Karger.

Dervin, B. (1989). Audience as listener and learner, teacher and confidante: The sense-making approach. In R. Rice and C. Atkin (eds.), *Public Communication Campaigns*, 2nd edition (pp. 67-86). Newbury Park, CA: Sage.

Deutsch, K. (1966). *Nationalism and social communication: An inquiry into the foundation of nationality*. Cambridge, MA: MIT Press.

DiMatteo, M. (1982). *Social psychology and medicine*. Cambridge, MA: Olgeschlager, Gunn, and Hain.

DiMatteo, M. (1979). A social psychological analysis of physician-patient rapport: Toward a science of the art of medicine. *Journal of Social Issues*, 35, 12-33.

Dissanayake, W. (1989). Intercultural communication as a focus of research. In S. King (ed.), *Human communication as a field of study*. Albany, NY: State University of New York Press.

Dreyfuss, I. (1986, June 4). Anybody listening? *APA Newswire*.

Ducanis, A., and Golin, A. (1979). *The interdisciplinary health care team: A handbook*. Germantown, MD: Aspens Systems Corporation.

Edgar, T., Hammond, S. L., and Freimuth, V. S. (1989). Mediated and interpersonal strategies for the prevention of AIDS. *AIDS and Public Policy Journal*, 4, 3-9.

Eichhorn, S. (1974). *Becoming: The actualization of individual differences in five student health teams*. Bronx, NY: Institute for Health Team Development.

Eiler, G. (1990). Focus on focus groups. *Marketing and Media Decisions*, 35, 51.

Ellis, B., Miller, K., and Given, C. (1989). Caregivers in home health care situations: Measurement and relations among critical concepts. *Health Communication*, 1, 207-225.

Elmore, G. (1981, April). *Integrating video technology and organizational communication*. Paper presented to the Indiana Speech Association conference, Indianapolis.

Emry, R., and Wiseman, R. (1985, November). *An intercultural understanding of ablebodied and disabled persons' communication*. Paper presented to the Speech Communication Association conference, Denver.

Enelow, A., and Swisher, S. (1972). *Interviewing and patient care*. New York: Oxford University Press.

Farley, M. J., and Stoner, M. (1989). The nurse executive and interdisciplinary team building. *Nursing Administration Quarterly*, 13, 24-30.

Fish, S. (1990). Therapeutic uses of the telephone: Crisis intervention vs. traditional therapy. In G. Gumpert and S. Fish, (eds.), *Talking with strangers: Mediated therapeutic communication*. Norwood, NJ: Ablex.

Fisher, B. A. (1974). *Small group decision making: Communication and process*. New York: McGraw-Hill.

Fisher, W. R. (1987). *Human communication as narration*. Columbia, SC: University of South Carolina Press.

Fisher, W. R. (1985). The narrative paradigm: An elaboration. *Communication Monographs*, 52, 347-367.

Fisher, W. R. (1984). Narration as a human communication paradigm: The case of public moral argument. *Communication Monographs*, 51, 1-22.

Flay, B. R. (1987). Mass media and smoking cessation: A critical review. *American Journal of Public Health*, 77, 153-160.

Flay, B. R. (1986). Mass-media linkages with school-based programs for drug abuse prevention. *Journal of School Health*, 56, 402-406.

Flay, B., and Burton, D. (1990). Effective mass communication strategies for health campaigns. In C. Atkin and L. Wallack (eds.), *Mass communication and public health* (pp. 129-148). Newbury Park, CA: Sage.

Flay, B. R., and Cook, T. (1981). Evaluation of mass media prevention campaigns. In R. Rice and W. Paisley (eds.), *Public communication campaigns*. Beverly Hills: Sage, 239-264.

Flay, B. R., DiTecco, D., and Schlegel, R. P. (1980). Mass media and health promotion: An analysis using an extended information processing model. *Health Education Quarterly*, 7, 127-147.

Flora, J., Maccoby, N., and Farquhar, J. (1989). Communication campaigns to prevent cardiovascular disease: The Stanford community studies. In R. Rice and C. Atkin (eds.), *Public Communication Campaigns*, 2nd edition (pp. 233-252). Newbury Park, CA: Sage.

Foley, R., and Sharf, B. (1981). The five interviewing techniques most frequently overlooked by primary care physicians. *Behavioral Medicine*, 11, 26-31.

Fowler, M. (1988). Nursing ethics committees. *Heart and Lung*, 17, 718-719.

Frank, L. (1961). Interprofessional communication. *American Journal of Public Health*, 51, 1798-1804.

Freidson, E. (1970). *Professional dominance: The social structure of medical care.* Chicago: Aldine Publications.

Freimuth, V. S. (1979). Assessing the readability of health education messages. *Public Health Reports*, 94, 568-570.

Freimuth, V. S., Stein, J. A., and Kean, T. J. (1989). *Searching for health information.* Philadelphia: University of Pennsylvania Press.

Froland, C., Brodsky, G., Olson, M., and Stewart, L. (1979). Social support and social adjustment: Implications for mental health professionals. *Community Mental Health Journal*, 15, 82-93.

Frost, J., and Wilmot, W. (1978). *Interpersonal conflict.* Dubuque, IA: William C. Brown.

Fuller, D., and Quesada, G. (1973). Communication in medical therapeutics. *Journal of Communication*, 23, 361-370.

Geist, P., and Hardesty, M. (1990). Reliable, silent, hysterical, or assured: Physicians assess patient cues in their medical decision making. *Health Communication*, 69-90.

Gibb, J. (1961). Defensive communication. *Journal of Communication*, 11, 141-148.

Gilligan, C. (1982). *In a different voice.* Cambridge: Harvard University Press.

Gochman, D. (1969). Measuring health-relevant expectancies. *Psychological Reports*, 24, 880-886.

Goffman, E. (1963). *Stigma: Notes on the management of spoiled identity.* Englewood Cliffs, NJ: Spectrum.

Gorney, M. (1988). *The Doctors' Company risk management guide.* Santa Monica, CA: The Doctors' Company, Risk Management Committee.

Gottlieb, B. (1981). *Social networks and social support.* Beverly Hills, CA: Sage.

Gouran, D. (1974). Perspectives on the study of leadership: Its present and its future. *Quarterly Journal of Speech*, 60, 376-381.

Greenbaum, T. (1989). Groups: Helpful or harmful? *Bank Marketing*, 21, 26-27.

Greenfield, S., Kaplan, S., and Ware, J. (1985). Expanding patient involvement in care: Effects on patient outcomes. *Annals of Internal Medicine*, 102, 520-528.

Grunig, J. E. (1989). Public, audiences, and market segments: Station principles for campaigns. In C. Salmon (ed.), *Information campaigns: Balancing social values and social change* (pp. 189-228). Newbury Park, CA: Sage.

Gudykunst, W. (1989). Culture and the development of interpersonal relationships, In J. Anderson (ed.), *Communication Yearbook 12* (pp. 315-354). Newbury Park, CA: Sage.

Haakenson, R. (1977). A good talk: C.O.D.: Content, organization, and delivery. In B. Peterson, et al. (eds.), *Communication probes*. Chicago: Science Research Associates.

Hall, B. (1977). *Mtu ni afya: Tanzania's health campaign.* Washington, D.C.: Agency for International Development.

Hall, E. (1976). *Beyond culture.* Garden City, NY: Doubleday.

Hall, E. (1966). *The hidden dimension.* Garden City, NY: Doubleday.

Hall, E. (1959). *The silent language.* Garden City, NY: Doubleday.

Hardin, S., and Halaris, A. (1983). Nonverbal communication of patients and high and low empathy of nurses. *Journal of Psychosocial Nursing and Mental Health Services,* 21, 14-20.

Harlem, O. (1977). *Communication in medicine.* Paris: S. Karger.

Harrigan, J., and Rosenthal, R. (1986). Nonverbal aspects of empathy and rapport in physician-patient interaction. In P. Blanck, R. Buck, and R. Rosental (eds.), *Nonverbal communication in the clinical context* (pp. 36-73). University Park: Pennsylvania State University Press.

Hawkins, R., Day, T., Guztafson, D., Chewning, B., and Bosworth, K. (1982, May). *Using computer programs to provide health information to adolescents: BARNY.* Paper presented to the ICA conference, Boston.

Heimann-Ratain, G., Hanson, M., and Peregoy, S. M. (1985). The role of focus groups in designing a smoking prevention program. *Journal of School Health,* 55, 13-16.

Heineken, J. (1983). Treating the disconfirmed psychiatric patient. *Journal of Psychosocial Nursing and Mental Health Services,* 21, 21-25.

Heineken, J., and Roberts, F. (1983). Confirming not disconfirming: Communicating in a more positive manner. *American Journal of Maternal Child Nursing,* 8. 78-80.

Heiney, S., and Wells, L. (1989). Strategies for organizing and maintaining successful support groups. *Oncology Nursing Forum,* 16, 803-809.

Henderson, G., and Primeaux, M. (1981). *Transcultural health care.* Menlo Park, CA: Addison-Wesley.

Herlicky, C. (1970). Physician-patient rapport: A vital relationship. *Journal of the Medical Association of Alabama,* 40, 181.

Herscher, J. (March 2, 1991). New AIDS information campaign. *San Francisco Chronicle,* Section A, 24.

Hertz, P., and Stamps, P. (1977). Appointment-keeping behavior re-evaluated. *American Journal of Public Health,* 67, 1033-1036.

Hill, S. K. (1978). Health communication: Focus on interprofessional communication. *Communication Administration Bulletin,* 25, 31-36.

Hocker, J., and Wilmot, W. (1985). *Interpersonal conflict,* 2nd edition. Dubuque, IA: William C. Brown.

Hoppe, S., and Heller, P. (1975). Alienation, familism, and the utilization of health services by Mexican-Americans. *Journal of Health and Social Behavior,* 16, 304-314.

House, R. (1970). Role conflict and multiple authority in complex organizations. *California Management Review,* 12, 53-60.

Hughey, J., Norton, R., Edgar, T., and Adamson, B. (1986, November). An explanatory analysis of the media coverage of AIDS and men at risk. Paper presented to the Speech Communication Association conference, Chicago.

Hulka, B., Cassel, J., and Kupper, L. (1976). Communication compliance, and concordance between physicians and patients with prescribed medications. *American Journal of Public Health*, 66, 847-853.

Hulka, B., Kupper, L., and Cassel, J. (1975). Medication use and misuse: Physician-patient discrepancies. *Journal of Chronic Diseases*, 28, 7-21.

Humphris, D. (1988). Team working — breaking down the barriers. *Nursing*, 3, 999-1005.

Illich, I., Zola, I., McKnight, J., Caplan, J., and Shaiken, H. (1977). *The disabling professions*. Salem, NH: Marion Boyers Press.

Jacobson, B., and Amos, A. (1985). *When smoke gets in your eyes: Cigarette advertising policy and coverage of smoking and health in women's magazines*. London: British Medical Association/Health Education Council.

Johnson, D., and Clarke, V. (1984). Part two, Quality circles: Developing quality of care. *Nursing Times*, 51, 36-37.

Jourard, S. (1964). *The transparent self*. Princeton, NJ: Van Nostrand Co.

Kalish, R., and Collier, K. (1981). *Exploring human values*. Monterey, CA: Brooks/Cole.

Kane, R., and Deuschle, K. (1967). Problems in doctor-patient communication. *Medical Care*, 5, 260-271.

Kaplan, B. (1985). Barriers to medical computing: History, diagnosis, and therapy for the medical computing lag. In G. Cohen (ed.), *Proceedings of the ninth annual symposium on computer applications in medical care*. Silver Spring, MD: IEEE/Computer Society Press, 400-404.

Kaufman, L. (1980). Prime-time nutrition. *Journal of Communication*, 30, 37-46.

Keelan, J., and Stokoe, S. (1983). Taking the stress out of OR communication. *AORN Journal*, 37, 847-853.

Kelly, F. (1972). Communication significance of therapist proxemic cues. *Journal of Consulting and Clinical Psychology*, 39, 345.

Kindig, D. (1975). Interdisciplinary education for primary health care team delivery. *Journal of Medical Education*, 50, 97-110.

Kisker, E. (1985). Teenagers talk about sex, pregnancy, and contraception. *Family Planning Perspectives*, 17, 83-90.

Kitson, A. (1987). A comparitive analysis of lay-caring and professional (nursing) caring relationships. *International Journal of Nursing Studies*, 24, 155-165.

Kleinman, A. (1988). *The illness narratives: Suffering, healing, and the human condition*. New York: Basic Books.

Knapp, M. (1978). *Nonverbal communication in human interaction*, 2nd edition. New York: Holt, Rinehart, and Winston.

Kohlberg, L. (1981). The philosophy of moral development. *Human Development*, 12, 93-120.

Korsch, B., and Negrete, V. (1972). Doctor-patient communication. *Scientific American*, 227, 66-74.

Korsch, B. M., Gozzi, E., and Francis, V. (1968). Gaps in doctor-patient communication. *Pediatrics*, 42, 855-871.

Kosa, J., and Zola, I. (eds.), (1975). *Poverty and health: A sociological analysis*. Cambridge, MA: Harvard University Press.

Kotler, P. (1975). *Marketing for Non-Profit Organizations*. Englewood Cliffs, NJ: Prentice-Hall.

Kotler, P. and Roberto, E. (1989). *Social marketing: Strategies for changing public behavior*. New York: Free Press.

Kreps, G. L. (1990a). *Organizational communication: Theory and practice*, 2nd edition. White Plains, NY: Longman.

Kreps, G. L. (1990b). A systematic analysis of health communication with the aged. In H. Giles, N. Coupland, and J. Wiemann (eds.), *Communication, health, and the elderly* (135-154). Fulbright Colloquium Series Number 8, Manchester, U.K.: University of Manchester Press.

Kreps, G.L. (1990c). Communication and health education. In E. B. Ray and L. Denohew (eds.), *Communication and health: Systems and applications* (pp. 187-203).

Kreps, G. L. (1990d). Stories as repositories of organizational intelligence: Implications for organizational development. In J. Anderson (ed.), *Communication Yearbook 13* (pp. 191-202). Newbury Park, CA: Sage.

Kreps, G. L. (1990, November). *The value of therapeutic communication in organizational life*. Paper presented to the Speech Communication Association conference, Chicago.

Kreps, G. L. (1989). Communicating about death. *Journal of Communication Therapy*, 4, 2-13.

Kreps, G. L. (1988a). The pervasive role of information in health and health care: Implications for health communication policy. In J. Anderson (ed.), *Communication Yearbook 11* (pp. 238-276).

Kreps, G. L. (1988b). Relational communication in health care. *The Southern Speech Communication Journal*, 53, 344-359.

Kreps, G. L. (1986a). *A relational analysis of the role of information in health and health care*. Paper presented to the Communicating with Patients conference, University of South Florida, Tampa.

Kreps, G. L. (1986b). Health communication and the elderly. *World Communication*, 15, 55-70.

Kreps, G. L. (1980). A field experimental test and revaluation of Weick's model of organizing. In D. Nimmo (ed.), *Communication Yearbook 4* (pp. 389-398). New Brunswick: NJ: Transaction.

Kreps, G. L., and Atkin, C. (1991). Current issues in health communication research. *American Behavioral Scientist*, 34, 648-651.

Kreps, G. L., and Maibach, E. W. (1991, May). *Communicating to prevent health risks*. Paper presented to the International Communication Association conference, Chicago.

Kubler-Ross, E. (1969). *On death and dying*. New York: MacMillan.

Lane, S. (1982). Communication and patient compliance. In L. Pettegrew (ed.), *Straight talk: Explorations in provider-patient interaction*. Louisville, KY: Humana Corporation.

Lane, S. (1983). Compliance, satisfaction, and physician-patient communication. In R. Bostrum (ed.), *Communication Yearbook 7* (pp. 772-799). Newbury Park, CA: Sage.

Larsen, K., and Smith, C. (1981). Assessment of nonverbal communication in the patient-physician interview. *Journal of Family Practice*, 12, 481-488.

Larson, C. E., and LaFasto, F. (1989). *Teamwork: What must go right/what can go wrong*. Newbury Park, CA: Sage.

Lawler, E. E., and Mohrman, S. A. (1985). Quality circles after the fad. *Harvard Business Review*, 63, 65-71.

Lefebvre, C., and Flora, J. (1988). Social marketing and public health intervention. *Health Education Quarterly*, 15, 299-315.

Lehman, M. (1986, September/October). Quality circles: Their place in health care. *Hospital Topics*, 15-19.

Levine-Ariff, J., and Groh, D. (1990). *Creating an ethical environment*. Baltimore, MD: William and Wilkins.

Levy, A., and Stokes, R. (1987). Effects of a health promotion advertising program on sales of "ready to eat" cereals. *Public Health Reports*, 102, 398-403.

Ley, P. (1982). Giving information to patients. In J. R. Eiser (ed.), *Social psychology and behavioral medicine* (pp. 339-374). London: John Wiley and Sons.

Lucaites, J. L., and Condit, C. M. (1985). Reconstructing narrative theory: A functional perspective. *Journal of Communication*, 35, 90-108.

Lum, R. (1987). The patient-counselor relationship in cross-cultural context. In B. Biesecker, P. Magyari, and N. Paul (eds.), *Strategies in genetic counseling: Religious, cultural, and ethnic influences on the counseling process* (pp. 133-143). New York: March of Dimes Birth Defects Foundation.

Mabry, E., and Barnes, R. (1980). *The dynamics of small group communication*. Englewood Cliffs, NJ: Prentice-Hall.

Maccoby, N., and Farquhar, J. (1975). Communication for health: Unselling heart disease. *Journal of Communication*, 25, 114-126.

Maccoby, N., and Solomon, D. S. (1981). Heart disease prevention: Community studies. In R. Rice and W. Paisley (eds.), *Public Communication Campaigns* (pp. 105-126). Beverly Hills, CA: Sage.

Madara, E. (1987, Fall). Supporting self-help: A clearinghouse perspective. *Journal of Social Policy*, 18, 28-29.

Mailhot, C., and Slezak, L. (1983). Nurse-physician committee eases tension in the OR. *Association of Operating Room Nursing Journal*, 38, 411-415.

Makris, P. (1983). Informatics in health-care delivery systems. *Information Age*, 5, 205-210.

Martiney, R. (1978). *Hispanic culture and health care — fact, fiction and folklore*. St. Louis: C.V. Mosby Company.

McCombs, M. E., and Shaw, D. L. (1972). The agenda-setting function of the media. *Public Opinion Quarterly*, 36, 176-188.

McElroy, A., and Townsend, P. K. (1989). *Medical anthropology*, 2nd edition. Boulder, CO: Westview Press.

McGuire, W. J. (1989). Theoretical foundations of campaigns. In R. Rice and C. Atkin (eds.), *Public communication campaigns*, 2nd edition (pp. 43-67). Newbury Park, CA: Sage.

McGrath, J. C. (1991). Evaluating national health communication campaigns. *American Behavioral Scientist*, 34, 653-665.

McIntosh, J. (1974). Process of communication, information seeking control associated with cancer: A selected review of the literature. *Social Science and Medicine*, 8, 167-187.

McLaughlin, J. (1975). The doctor shows. *Journal of Communication*, 25, 182-184.

McManus, J. (1989). Operation eyesight universal asset third world opthalmic teams. *Journal of Opthalmic Nursing and Technology*, 8, 236-238.

Mechanic, D. (1972). *Public expectations and health care: Essays on the changing organizations of health services*. New York: Wiley.

Melton, W. (1984, December 28). Controversial cancer victim dead at 13. *Reno-Gazette Journal*. Reno, NV, 22.

Mendelsohn, R. (1979). *Confessions of a medical heretic*. Chicago: Contemporary Books.

Mendelsohn, R. (1981). *Male practice: How doctors manipulate women*. Chicago: Contemporary Books.

Mendelson, M. (1974). *Tender loving greed*. New York: Knopps.

Milmoe, S., et al. (1967). The doctor's voice: Postdictor of successful referral of alcoholic patients. *Journal of Abnormal Psychology*, 72, 78-84.

Mintzberg, H. (1973). *The nature of managerial work*. New York: Harper and Row.

Mishler, E. G. (1984). *The discourse of medicine: Dialectic of medical interviews*. Norwood, NJ: Ablex.

Montagu, A. (1971). *Touching: The human significance of skin*. New York: Columbia University Press.

Moulder, P., Staal, A., and Grant, M. (1988). Making the interdisciplinary team work. *Rehabilitation Nursing*, 13, 338-339.

Myerhoff, B., and Larson, W. (1965). The doctor as cultural hero: The routinization of charisma. *Human Organization*, 24, 188-191.

Nagi, S. Z. (1975). Teamwork in health care in the United States: A sociological perspective. *The Milbank Memorial Fund Quarterly*, 53, 36.

National Cancer Institute. (1984). *Pretesting in health communications* (NIH Publication No. 84-143). Bethesda, MD. USDHHS.

Nelson, B. (1973). Study indicates which patients nurses don't like: The unpleasant, the long term, the mentally ill, the hypochondriacs, and the dying. *Modern Hospital*, 119, 70-72.

Nelson, R. (1981). What is the payoff in computerized appointment scheduling. *Medical Group Management*, (July, August), 18-21.

Nichols, R. (1957). *Are you listening?* New York: McGraw-Hill.

Nodding, N. (1984). *Caring*. Berkeley, CA: University of California Press.

Northouse, P. (1977). Predictors of empathic ability in an organizational setting. *Human Communication Research*, 3, 176-178.

O'Donnell, M. P., and Ainsworth, T. H. (eds). (1984). *Health promotion in the workplace*. New York: John Wiley and Sons.

O'Hair, D., Kreps, G. L., and Frey, L. (1990). Conceptual issues. In D. O'Hair and G. L. Kreps (eds.), *Applied communication theory and research* (pp. 3-22). Hillsdale, NJ: Erlbaum.

Pacanowsky, M., and O'Donnell-Trujillo, N. (1982). Communication and organizational cultures. *Western Journal of Speech Communication*, 41, 115-130.

Page, W. (1980). Rhetoritherapy vs. behavior therapy: Issues and evidence. *Communication Education*, 29, 95-104.

Palleschi, P., and Heim, P. (1980). The hidden barriers to team building. *Training and Development Journal*, 34, 14-18.

Park, B., and Bashshur, R. (1975). Some implications of telemedicine. *Journal of Communication*, 25, 161-166.

Payer, L. (1988). *Medicine and culture*. New York: Penguin Books.

Pelletier, L. (1983). Interpersonal communications task group. *Journal of Psychosocial Nursing and Mental Health Services*, 21, 33-75, 91.

Perrow, C. (1965). Hospitals, technology, structure and goals. In J. March (ed.), *Handbook of organizations* (pp. 910-971). Chicago: Rand McNally.

Pettegrew, L. (1977). An investigation of therapeutic communication style. In B. Ruben (ed.), *Communication Yearbook 1* (593-604). New Brunswick, NJ: Transaction.

Petty, R. E., and Cacioppo, J. T. (1981). *Attitudes and persuasion: Classic and contemporary approaches*. Dubuque, IA: William C. Brown.

Pfeffer, J. (1973). Size, composition and function of hospital boards of directors: A study of organization-environment linkage. *Administrative Science Quarterly*, 18, 449-461.

Pfeffer, J., and Salancik, G. (1977). Organizational context and the characteristics and tenure of hospital administrators. *Academy of Management Journal*, 20, 74-88.

Plachy, R. (1973, May). You theory x, me theory y! *Modern Hospital*, 120, 73-78.

Piuchman, M. (1978). *Human communication: The matrix of nursing*. New York: McGraw-Hill.

Portnoy, B., Anderson, D. M., and Eriksen, M. P. (1989). Application of diffusion theory to health promotion research. *Family and Community Health*, 12 (3), 63-71.

Presidents Commission for the Study of Ethical Problems in Medicine and Biomedical and Behavioral Research. (1982). *Making health care decisions: The ethical and legal implications of informed consent in the patient-practitioner relationship* (Vols. 1 and 2). Washington, DC: Government Printing Office.

Purtilo, R. (1978). *Health professional/patient interaction*. Philadelphia: W. B. Saunders.

Putnam, L. (1982). Procedural messages and small group work climates: A lag sequential analysis. In M. Burgoon (ed.), *Communication Yearbook 5* (pp. 331-350). New Brunswick, NJ: Transaction.

Quesada, G., and Heller, R. (1977). Sociolcultural barriers to medical care among Mexican-Americans in Texas. *Medical Care*, 15, 93-101.

Rawls, J. (1971) *A theory of justice*. Cambridge, MA: Harvard University Press.

Ray, E. B. (1983). Job burnout from a communication perspective. In R. Bostrum (ed.), *Communication Yearbook 7* (738-755). Newbury Park, CA: Sage.

Ray, E. B., and Miller, K. (1990). Communication in health care organizations. In E. B. Ray and L. Donohew (eds.), *Communication and health: Systems and applications* (92-107). Hillsdale, NJ: Erlbaum.

Reardon, K. K. (1988). The role of persuasion in health promotion and disease prevention: A review and commentary. In J. A. Anderson (ed.), *Communication Yearbook 11* (pp. 277-297). Newbury Park, CA: Sage.

Reardon, K. K., and Rogers, E. M. (1988). Interpersonal versus mass communication: A false dichotomy. *Human Communication Research,* 15, 284-303.

Reich, W. T. (1985). Moral absurdities in critical care medicine: Commentary on a parable. In J. C. Moskop and L. Kopelaan (eds.), *Ethical and critical care medicine* (pp. 11-21). Dordrecht, Holland: D. Reidel.

Relman, A. A. (1982). Encouraging the practice of preventive medicine and health promotion. *Public Health Reports,* 97, 216-219.

Ribble, D. (1989). Psychosocial support groups for people with HIV infection and AIDS. *Holistic Nursing Practice,* 3, 52-62.

Richman, J. M. (1989). Social support for hospice teams. Home Healthcare Nurse, 7, 8-38.

Robson, M. (1984). Quality circles, four: The American experience. *Nursing Times,* 51, 32.

Rogers, C. R. (ed.), (1967). *The therapeutic relationship and its impact.* Madison, WI: University of Wisconsin Press.

Rogers, E. M. (1983). *Diffusion of innovations.* New York: Free Press.

Rogers, E. M., and Agarwala-Rogers, R. (1976). *Communication in organizations.* New York: Free Press.

Rogers, E. M., and Kinkaid, D. (1981). *Communication networks: Toward a new paradigm for research.* New York: Free Press.

Rogers, E. M., and Storey, J. D. (1987). Communication campaigns. In C. Berger and S. Chafee (eds.), *Handbook of communication science.* Newbury Park, CA: Sage.

Rosen, G. (1976). *Preventive medicine in the United States 1900-1975.* New York: Prodist, 1976.

Ross, J. (1986). *Handbook for hospital ethics committees.* Chicago: American Hospital Publishing Company.

Rossiter, C. (1975). Defining therapeutic communication. *Journal of Communication,* 25, 127-130.

Rossiter, C., and Pearce, N. (1975). *Communicating personally.* Indianapolis: Bobbs-Merrill.

Roter, D., and Hall, J. (1986, October). *Meta analysis of correlates of provider behavior: A contribution to a theory of effective provider behavior.* Paper presented to the international conference on doctor-patient communication, University of Western Ontario, London, Ontario.

Roth, J. (1957). Ritual and magic in the control of contagion. *American Sociological Review,* 23, 311-312.

Rubinson, L., and Alles, W. F. (1984, 1988 reissue). *Health education: Foundations for the future.* Prospect Heights, IL: Waveland Press.

Ruddick, S. (1989). *Maternal thinking: Toward a politics of peace*. Boston: Beacon Press.

Ruesch, J. (1957). *Disturbed communication*. New York: W.W. Norton.

Salmond, S. (1990). In hospital case management. *Orthodpaedic Nursing, 9*, 38-40.

Samovar, L., and Porter, R. (1991). *Understanding intercultural communication*, 6th edition. Belmont, CA: Wadsworth.

Samovar, L., Porter, R., and Jain, N. (1981). *Understanding intercultural communication*. Belmont, CA.: Wadsworth.

Sethee, U. (1967). Verbal responses of nurses to patients in emotion-laden situations in public health nursing. *Nursing Research, 16*, 365-368.

Sharf, B. F. (1990) Physician-patient communication as interpersonal rhetoric: A narrative approach. *Health Communication, 2*, 217-231.

Simoni, J., and Ball, R. (1975). Can we learn from medicine hucksters? *Journal of Communication, 25*, 174-181.

Simoni, J. J., Vargas, L. A., and Casillas, L. (1982, May). *Medicine showmen and the communication of health information*. Paper presented to the International Communication Association conference, Boston.

Sitaram, K., and Cogdell, R. (1976). *Foundations of intercultural communication*. Columbus, OH: Charles E. Merrill.

Slack, W., Hicks, W., Reed, C., and VanCura, L. (1966). A computer-based medical history. *New England Journal of Medicine, 274*, 194-198.

Smith, D. H. (1987). Telling stories as a way of doing ethics. *Journal of the Florida Medical Association, 74*, 581-588.

Smith, R. (1976). Doctors and patients. Boise, ID: Syms-York.

Sobel, J., and Brown, J. (1982, May). *Public health agenda-setting: Evaluation of a cardiovascular risk-reduction campaign*. Paper presented to the International Communication Association conference, Boston.

Solomon, D. S. (1984). Social marketing and community health promotion: The Stanford heart disease prevention project. In L. Fredericksen, L. Salomon, and K. Brehony (eds.), *Marketing health behavior: Principles, techniques, and applications*. New York: Plenum Press, 115-135.

Solomon, D. S. (1989). A social marketing perspective on communication campaigns. In R. Rice and C. Atkin (eds.), *Public communication campaigns* (pp. 87-104). Newbury Park, CA: Sage.

Speedling, E., and Rose, D. (1985). Building an effective doctor-patient relationship: From patient satisfaction to patient participation. *Social Science and Medicine, 21*, 115-120.

Starosta, W. (1989). Ceteris paribus in the global village: A research agenda for intercultural communication theory building. In J. Anderson (ed.), *Communication Yearbook 12* (pp. 310-314). Newbury Park, CA: Sage.

Starr, P. (1982). *The social transformation of American medicine*. New York: Basic Books.

Stein, H. (1990). *American medicine as culture*. Boulder, CO: Westview Press.

Stewart, C., and Cash, W. (1978). *Interviewing principles and practices*, 2nd edition. Dubuque, IA: William C. Brown.

Stewart, M., and Roter, D. (eds.), (1989). *Communicating with medical patients.* Newbury Park, CA: Sage.

Stohl, C. (1986). Quality circles and changing patterns of communication. In M. McLaughlin (ed.), *Communication Yearbook 9* (pp. 511-531). Beverly Hills, CA: Sage.

Stohl, C. (1987). Bridging the parrallel organization: A study of quality circle effectiveness. In M. McLaughlin (ed.), *Communication Yearbook 10* (pp. 416-430). Newbury Park, CA: Sage.

Stone, G. (1979). Patient compliance and the role of the expert. *Journal of Social Issues, 35,* 34-59.

Street, R., and Wiemann, J. (1987). Patients' satisfaction with physicians' interpersonal involvement, expressiveness, and dominance. In M. McLaughlin (ed.), *Communication Yearbook 10* (pp. 591-612). Newbury Park, CA: Sage.

Talento, B., and Crocket-McKeever, L. (1983). Improving interviewing techniques. *Nursing Outlook, 31,* 234-235.

Tannen, D. (1990). *You just don't understand me.* New York: William Morrow and Company.

Thompson, P. (1982). *Quality circles: How to make them work in America.* New York: AMACOM.

Thornton, B. C. (1988). Blowing the whistle. *California Nursing Review, 10,* 24-27.

Thornton, B. C. (1978). Health care teams and multimethodological research. In B. Ruben (ed.), *Communication Yearbook 2* (pp. 538-553). New Brunswick, NJ: Transaction.

Thornton, B. C., McCoy, E., and Baldwin, D. (1980). Role relationships on interdisciplinary health care teams. In D. Baldwin, B. Rowley, and V. Williams (eds.), *Interdisciplinary health care teams in teaching and practice.* Reno, NV: New Health Perspectives.

Thornton, B. C., Page, P., and Dangott, L. (1982). Communication with patients regarding pain and anxiety. *The Dental Assistant, 51,* 22-23.

Tinello-Biddle, N. (1986). Quality circles: A management strategy that works. *Nursing Success Today, 3,* 9-11.

Tones, B. K. (1986). Health education and the ideology of health promotion: A review of alternative approaches. *Health Education Research, 1,* 3-12.

Toseland, R., Palmer-Ganeles, J., and Chapman, D. (1986, January/February). Teamwork in psychiatric settings. *Social Work,* 46-52.

Trauth, D., and Huffman, J. (1986, May). *Regulation of alcoholic beverage advertising: Its present status and future directions.* Paper presented at the International Communication Association conference, Chicago.

Tripp-Reimer, T., and Afifi, L. (1989). Cross cultural perspectives on patient teaching. *Nursing Clinics of North America, 24,* 613-622.

Truax, C., and Carkhuff, R. (1967). *Toward effective counseling and psychotherapy: Training and practice.* Chicago: Aldine.

Udry, J. (1972). Can mass media advertising increase contraceptive use? *Family Planning Perspectives, 4,* 37-44.

U.S. Department of Health and Human Services. (1989a). *Making health communication programs work* (NIH Publication No 89-1493). Bethesda, MD: NIH.

U.S. Department of Health and Human Services. (1989b). *Reducing the health consequences of smoking: Twenty-five years of progress.* Public Health Service, Centers for Disease Control, publication No. (CDC) 89-8411.

U.S. Senate Special Committee on Aging, Subcommittee on Long Term Care. (1974). *Nursing home care in the United States, failure in public policy: Introductory report.* Washington, D.C.: USGPO.

U.S. Senate Special Committee on Aging, Subcommittee on Long Term Care. (1975). *Nursing home care in the United States, failure in public policy: Introductory report and nine supporting papers.* Washington, D.C.: USGPO.

Vargas, M. (1987). Tradition of nontradition — our cultural blind spot. In B. Biesecker, P. Magyari and N. Paul (eds.), *Strategies in genetic counseling: Religious, cultural, and ethnic influences on the counseling process* (pp. 122-132). New York: March of Dimes Birth Defects Foundation.

Waitzkin, H., and Stoekle, J. (1976). Information control and the micropolitics of health care: Summary of an ongoing research project. *Social Science and Medicine, 10,* 263-276.

Walker, H. (1973). Communication and the American health care problem. *Journal of Communication, 23,* 349-360.

Wallace, R., and Benson, H. (1972). The physiology of meditation. *Scientific American, 226,* 84-90.

Wallack, L. M. (1981). Mass media campaigns: The odds against finding behavior change. *Health Education Quarterly, 8,* 209-260.

Wallack, L. M. (1990). Improving health promotion: Media advocacy and social marketing approaches. In C. Atkin and L. Wallack (eds.), *Mass communication and public health* (pp. 147-163). Newbury Park, CA: Sage.

Wandelt, M., Pierce, P., and Widdowson, R. (1981). Why nurses leave nursing and what can be done about it. *American Journal of Nursing, 81,* 72-77.

Watson, W. (1975). The meanings of touch: Geriatric nursing. *Journal of Communication, 25,* 104-112.

Watzlawick, P. (1963). A review of the double bind theory. *Family Process, 2.* 132-153.

Watzlawick, P., Beavin, J., and Jackson, D. (1967). *Pragmatics of human communication.* New York: W.W. Norton.

Watson, W. (1970). Body image and staff-to-resident deportment in a home for the aged. *Aging and Human Development, 1,* 345-359.

Weed, L. (1971). *Medical records, medical education and patient care: The problem-oriented record as a basic tool,* 5th edition. Cleveland: The Press of Case Western Reserve University.

Weick, K. (1979). *The social psychology of organizing,* 2nd edition. Reading, MA: Addison-Wesley.

Weston, W. W., and Brown, J. B. (1989). The importance of patients' beliefs. M. Stewart and D. Roter (eds.), *Communication with medical patients* (pp. 77-85). Newbury park, CA: Sage.

White, E. (1974). Health and the black person: An annotated bibliography. *American Journal of Nursing, 74,* 1839-1841.

White, M. (1990). Law and ethics law and medicine: An overview. In J. Fletcher (ed.), *Basic clinical ethics and health care law.* Charlottesville, VA: Ibis Publishing.

Wiesenfeld, A., and Weiss, H. (1979). Hairdressers and helping: Influencing the behavior of informal caregivers. *Professional Psychology,* 10, 786-792.

Wise, W., Beckhard, R., Rubin, I., and Kyte, A. (1974). *Making health teams work.* Cambridge, MA: Ballinger.

Witte, K. (1991). The role of culture in health and diseases. In L. Samovar and R. Porter (eds.), *Intercultural communication: A reader,* 6th edition (pp. 199-207). Belmont, CA: Wadsworth.

Wolf, G. (1981). Nursing turnover: Some causes and solutions. *Nursing Outlook,* April, 233-236.

Woods, D. (1975). Talking to people is a doctor game that doctors don't play, *Canadian Medical Association Journal,* 113, 1105-1106.

Zola, I. (1963). Problems of communication, diagnosis, and patient care: The interplay of patient, physician and clinic organization. *Journal of Medical Education,* 38, 829-838.

Name Index

Subject Index